MW01223630

HUMAN BECOMING:
A GUIDE TO SOUL-CENTERED LIVING

R. M. LAMB PH.D.

Cittam Futures Inc.
Vancouver, B.C.

Front Cover Photograph: Gillian McFarlane
Cover Quote: Sri Aurobindo. From Aurobindo Ghose, Savitri (Pondicherry, India: Sri Aurobindo Ashram), 2005, p. 363.

ISBN: 978-0992120108
(CIP data available on request)

Published by Cittam Futures Inc. Vancouver, B.C.

www.cittamfutures.com

Our Vision: Seeking the spirit of natural healing from within.
Our Mission: Building Health—Creating Futures.
Our programs are national and international: Individuals who would like to arrange corporate, group, self-help, or presentations or programs based on the CITTAM Model for Integral Healing contact, our website. Our consciousness-based offerings are aimed at self-empowerment and the return of inner wisdom.

Disclaimer: *The content including the integral reflections outlined in this text is designed to be educational. If you experience anxiety or stress, please seek the assistance of your medical practitioner and only do these reflections under the guidance of a healthcare professional; these integral reflections are best considered an educational adjunct to conventional and complementary integrative health care. The appropriate medical authorities should be consulted for diagnosis and treatment of medical or psychological conditions. The author and publishers are in no way liable for the use or misuse of the information.*

HUMAN BECOMING:
A GUIDE TO SOUL-CENTERED LIVING

"Satellites of her sun they moved unable to forgo her light..."

Sri Aurobindo

List of Illustrations

All illustrations and charts copyright R.M. Lamb

CONTENTS

ACKNOWLEDGEMENTS

Human Becoming is dedicated to the Integrative Energy Healing practitioners and Advanced Integrative Healing practitioners who volunteered as interns in various research and educational projects featuring new dimensions of integral health care; to the students whose questions brought us all to a deeper understanding; to all the clients who have attended our supervised clinics and returned to tell of us the benefits; to Anna M. Fitzpatrick for her excellent editing suggestions, Doug Hilton for his image designs, Gillian McFarlane for the front cover photograph, and Allison James for the cover and image designs; to Julia (pseudonym) for her story; to Professor Arabinda Basu and Dr. Larry Seidlitz, my mentors and Sri Aurobindo scholars residing in India; to my husband who is capable of presenting diverse worldviews; and to my children and their children whose views and values I hope will uphold unity in diversity.

FOREWORD

This work is a beautiful synthesis of several traditions, especially Integral Yoga and Integrative Energy Healing, the latter a particular form of biofield healing, also known as subtle energy healing. The term "integral" has become very popular and is used as an adjective in various theories, practices, programs and institutions, highlighting their synthesis of East-West, ancient-modern, material-spiritual and/or scientific-mystical traditions. One of the important forerunners of this movement was Sri Aurobindo (1872-1950), the Cambridge- educated modern mystic of India, who developed Integral Yoga, and what are sometimes referred to as Integral Philosophy and Integral Yoga Psychology as its intellectual supports or elaborations. It is not necessary to introduce this complex system of thought here—Ruth explains that admirably in the book itself— but it may be useful to give some biographical context. At Cambridge, Sri Aurobindo was a first-class classics scholar, exploring the roots of Western civilization. When he returned to India he learned Sanskrit and dug into the roots of Indian civilization, while also immersing himself in various modern European and Indian literatures. He also had a short but influential career as a leader of the Indian Independence Movement—the first to put forth the ideal of Independence prominently before the mind of the Indian people through his political writings, as well as to establish it as a political force in the Indian Congress. It was during his imprisonment for a year while undergoing trial for sedition that his developing spiritual experiences assumed higher and ever-widening dimensions— permeating, uplifting, and transforming his entire outer life. After his acquittal, he re-entered politics briefly, but then shifted his focus to his spiritual work, which would absorb him for the last 40 years of his life.

He was soon joined in this spiritual work by Mirra Alfassa (1879-1973), a French occultist and artist with Egyptian ancestry, who later became known as the Mother. Along with her husband, they started a monthly philosophical magazine, the Arya, which was to be "a systematic study of the highest problems of existence" and "a vast synthesis of knowledge, harmonizing the diverse religious traditions of humanity occidental as well as oriental." But after some months, WWI broke out and the Mother and her husband had to leave India, while Sri Aurobindo took up the magazine and used it as a vehicle to publish in installments much of his massive 35 volume corpus, working on as many as six major works simultaneously along with shorter essays. Six years later, soon after the war ended, the magazine ceased and the Mother returned and joined him as his spiritual collaborator. She eventually took charge of the development of the Ashram, the community of disciples that began to gather around them. She took charge not only of the development of its outer infrastructure which eventually grew into something like a small town, but also of the spiritual guidance and development of the disciples. On his side, Sri Aurobindo retired to his Ashram room to focus on his inner spiritual work, while keeping up an active, at times daily correspondence with the disciples, as well as providing his spiritual influence and support. The Mother interacted with the disciples daily, initiated various cottage industries and departments to support the Ashram, started a school for the growing number of children, acquired lands and buildings, managed the whole affair, and poured her spiritual influences on all around her. Sri Aurobindo's writing continued during this period, and the Mother's own recorded talks, messages, and writings also eventually assumed a mass of many volumes. After Sri Aurobindo's passing, the Mother continued the inner spiritual work and the outer work solitarily. At the age of 90, she founded the experimental city of Auroville, dedicated to human unity, about 10 km from the Ashram; 44 years later both the Ashram and Auroville are vibrant communities working to manifest their spiritual ideals in collective living.

Ruth's initial entry into this subject was through nursing. In her dissertation for a Ph.D. in Transformative Learning and Change at the California Institute of Integral Studies, on which this work is largely based, Ruth explains that one day, shortly after her graduation from Nursing School, she was confronted with the limitations of the traditional allopathic medical model and the realities of subtle dimensions of existence. A patient in intensive care had a cardiac arrest. As the nurse in charge, she called the alert code, applied cardiac defibrillation while other nurses initiated other aspects of the cardiac arrest procedure, all prior to the arrival of the on-call physician. The patient stabilized and regained consciousness. After a short time, while checking on him, he shyly confided to her that during the arrest, he had seen and heard them working on him from a place near the ceiling in the far corner of the room. Although not a part of the allopathic world-view, she accepted his experience at face- value. She shared it with her colleague, who replied with a similar experience that she once had but had never told to anyone. Ruth later found literature references to similar experiences of patients not shared with their physicians because of the embarrassment of not being believed and taken seriously. While not elaborated on in this book, there are important implications of this work for the limitations of the allopathic model, and for the advocacy and development of alternative approaches to medicine.

As she explained in her dissertation, Ruth began to intuitively sense the energy fields of her patients. She learned to stand quietly beside her patients and sense whether they would be stable during that shift, or if she should be especially vigilant to watch for signs of deterioration. Time and again her intuitions proved correct. Later she studied

Traditional Chinese Medicine and learned about chi, the subtle energy that supports the body. Before long she was studying, then teaching Therapeutic Touch and Healing Touch, two forms of subtle energy healing developed by nurses. Later she completed the four year Brennan Healing Science curriculum when it was taught out of New York. Still later she was drawn to North India to study related Tibetan Buddhist principles of healing and to teach a three year synthesis program including Tibetan Buddhism and biofield healing to Tibetan Buddhist nuns in Dharamsala. Finally, after much reading of Sri Aurobino's work, she travelled to South India to study the spiritual philosophy and yoga of Sri Aurobindo and its relations to subtle energy healing. Now she is training practitioners of Advanced Integrative Energy Healing at a college in British Columbia, and working as an international consultant in this field. She recently helped establish a healing center near Auroville where this treatment is being used along with other natural methods, catering especially to the local Tamil villagers.

It should be noted that this work is integrative not only in the sense of synthesizing Sri Aurobindo's and the Mother's Integral Yoga, Philosophy, and Psychology with subtle energy healing, but also, in linking all of these with the treatment of drug addiction and its accompanying severe psychological distress. Although not discussed in this book, in her dissertation Ruth utilized a research method called grounded theory, in which the researcher immerses herself in the real-life healing phenomenon being examined, and seeks for underlying patterns such that an organizing and explanatory theory emerges from the data. In Ruth's study, there were really two simultaneous approaches to the development of her theoretical explanations— the grounded theory that emerged from her immersion in the interview and clinical data collected from individuals with addictions and their subtle energy practitioners, and its synthesis with Sri Aurobindo's and the Mother's system of spiritual thought. As such, we could say that Ruth presents here the theory of Integral Yoga Psychology which is grounded in the practice of healing severe psychological distress associated with drug addiction, typically based in childhood abuse and trauma. This clientele may be unique with important differences from healthy adults, but it is also true that they are simply human beings who happen to be under severe stress with impacts on their mental, emotional, physical and subtle energy systems more clearly obvious. Thus, we may expect that although they would exhibit more powerful energy disruptions, and possibly more dramatic changes from subtle energy treatments than healthy adults, the underlying processes at work would likely be similar and applicable to us all.

This work weaves these different threads together into a rich tapestry which reveals to us dimensions of our own existence that we may not have suspected. As Ruth quotes Sri Aurobindo as saying, "It is only when we go behind, below, above into the hidden stretches of our being that we can know it..." She leads us into these hidden stretches first through the spiritual psychology of Sri Aurobindo and the Mother, and then more vividly through the reported experiences of the clients and subtle energy practitioners, often in their own words, which illustrate the psychological concepts. At the same time, this is not a static picture of the psychological experience of her research participants, but a fascinating story of their dynamic journey of inner self-finding, a journey on which we are all travelers.

Larry Seidlitz, PhD
Vice President, Student Affairs
Sri Aurobindo Centre for Advanced Research
Pondicherry, Tamil Nadu, India

INTRODUCTION

As the philosopher-seer Sri Aurobindo articulates, yoga nurtures the sacred unfolding of human becoming. It acknowledges the individual in the moment and encourages further development of consciousness from the view of a complex and astoundingly beautiful system that builds light, knowledge, and truth—and moreover, sets them into daily life as a living practice. As M. P. Pandit (1999) expresses well, Integral yoga places the focus on integration "in such a way that all its diverse powers in varying stages of growth are coordinated and forged together so as to leave out no element of the scheme" (p. 5). This complexity includes both external and internal life- activity and the development of the capacities and potentialities that lie within each individual such that the soul or sacredness within can emerge and claim its rightful freedom. This integral view of yoga supports the notion that as consciousness on the planet evolves, so does a yoga that concerns itself with the awakening and activating of consciousness.

At this time, as a planet we are immersed in information- overload, strife, and considerable chaotic activity on many dimensions. It is easy to be lost in everyday activities, and even easier to automatically become-the-activity: it is easy to be one- dimensional, effective, and efficient from a more physical and outer-consciousness perspective.

Only when we decide to stand back from the bustle of daily activity can something else come forward. In the core of the experience of stillness or strife, a luminous knowing, an eternal awareness, and an unlimited sense of something greater and impactful enters unexpectedly and remains in one's memory. Then it is possible—if there is time to reflect and a small witness-consciousness to 'hold' the experience—that a seeker may be born. The inner longing to stand back from the limiting circumstances of a bustling life can initiate a humble search inward to deeper layers and multiple dimensions, a search which leads to mystic teachings from the world's great cultures. Stories from the world's great traditions tell of the 'moment' that stops the ordinary and introduces the extraordinary, and thereby births the seeker; in Integral yoga it is the journey that uncovers the centre of divinity deep within. This centre and all that sustains it is seen as absolute Consciousness, Force, Energy, Light, and Information, and beyond, to Bliss, in the yoga of Sri Aurobindo. The route requires a change of consciousness, the opening of new doors of perception, and faith and belief in the grand scheme of a universal order far too astoundingly profound to grasp from any one viewpoint. With these tools acquired, an inner quest begins that elicits inner and outer coherence, potentially straightens relationships, and often renews one's sense of life-purpose or dharma.

The journey is one of soul and Light, and the evolution of Consciousness whereby the point of reference initially works to strengthen the ego-self to gain healthy egoic wisdom such that a new Beyond-ego state of development can be slowly formulated. The tapasya or work of the soul brings many challenges and much delight. The spiritual sadhana or inner aspiration for a life that includes more depth, sustenance, hope, and faith interweaves with the sacredness inherent in the soul of each being. 'Life' is renewed—the mystical side reborn. Moreover, for those with a love of science, the yogic science of Integral yoga has much to offer as it interweaves the rational and suprarational.

This book is an offering of and for the teachings of Sri Aurobindo and the Mother. The ideas herein follow years of serious study of Integral yoga and many trips to India to the Sri Aurobindo Ashram in Pondicherry and to Auroville, places steeped in the practices and teachings of Integral yoga where I studied with scholars and yogis of this great tradition.

The teachings as I have understood them became curriculum threads in an integrative healing program established in Vancouver, B.C., Canada in 1998 (Currently the Advanced Integrative Energy Healing Program). Offered through an academic and healthcare delivery system, the program combines science, inner work, awareness-based dialogue, professional practice, and supervised clinical biofield healing in healthcare delivery settings. The students and graduates of this certification program are, to my view, among the leaders in the new paradigm energy-based biofield health care of the future—a health care that hopefully will integrate many respected healing traditions. Only then will we have health promotion and enhancement for all that is affordable, appropriately effective, and self-empowering. Our success in clinical settings led to my doctoral work linking the advanced integrative healing our students were studying to Sri Aurobindo's Integral yoga. The outcome of this clinical grounded theory research is published in the text Healing as Yoga Sadhana (Lamb, 2010) or healing as the work of the soul. The text you hold now takes the next step in expanding and deepening the theory by linking quotes from my original research with the next phase of development: As discussed in this book, the Integral yoga view of consciousness as perceived through my current lens can be utilized for processes that sustain human becoming.

Centered on activating soul-centered consciousness —a consciousness that, from a multidimensional perspective, is situated deep in the energy of the heart— Integral yoga has a vast literature. Nominated for the Nobel prize in Literature in 1950 (the year he died), Sri Aurobindo has written volumes, and the Mother of the Sri Aurobindo Ashram, Mirra Alfassa has also written volumes, as have numerous highly skilled yogis and scholars over the span of Sri Aurobindo's and the Mother's lifetimes. The writing is ongoing. This text addresses an area that has been less well developed, bringing the teachings forward in conjunction with pragmatic wellness practices that are congruent today and are aimed at the development of self and soul and the process of human becoming. Working with clients and adult learners who wish to become new-paradigm practitioners led me to my own doctoral work, years after my initial RN, BA majoring in ancient philosophy, and MScN in nursing. To me personally, healing and learning go hand-in-hand as a sadhana of life, and the sadhana or practice of soul links inexorably with tapasya—the work of healing and learning and growing and evolving toward the noetic human, the next step in the human evolutionary process.

This text is presented in three parts, and in places incorporates integral practices from the Stations of Life Integral Healing model (see website for more information). *Part One: Yoga of Self and Soul* outlines a set of basic teachings that sustain the yoga of self and soul as I understand them from the work of Sri Aurobindo, the Mother, and other scholars of this tradition. Each chapter builds sophistication, taking us to the core of the Integral yoga teachings, and pragmatically personalizes the process by providing focused Integral Reflection questions or exercises and experiences designed as practices.

Part Two: Integral Dimensions of Consciousness examines consciousness, presence, and awareness from a multilayered integral view. We ask: What are we truly, behind all appearances? How do Consciousness, Light, Force, Energy, and Information configure within the human condition? A modern convergence of Western science and Eastern spirituality presents ideas on reality and its dimensions that are well supported in Integral yoga. These ideas, explored through yogic theory and practices, include developing a multilayered awareness of body consciousness that includes self-inquiry, heart-work, silence, sacred dialogue, and the renewal of faith. Doors open to understanding, integration, and action.

Part Three: Human Becoming continues to integrate

new Western science concepts with Integral yoga, overlaying processes for becoming that elicit and nurture the heart of the individual, the community, and the globe. The Path of Return from sadhana to soul is outlined with some of the main tenets reiterated. These are linked to ideas of rebirth and karma in ways that revisit human becoming and encourage individuals to light the flame of inquiry.

More specifically, Part One consists of chapters one through six. Chapter One focuses on the idea of oneness and consciousness, looking behind appearances for the underlying Oneness and using tools of consciousness-expansion to organize this consciousness-targeted worldview. Chapter Two outlines Sri Aurobindo's unique view of the evolution and involution of consciousness, discussing growth in awareness and its converse, dissolution into more automatic and trance-like ways of being. When combined with the specific practices presented, these teachings can be applied within the context of daily life and personal processes. Chapter Three speaks to the need to centralize the ego from an outer and inner being perspective before attempting a yoga of consciousness; Chapter Four discusses ways in which the ego is fractured and aspects of dissolution and traumas that veil wholeness. This chapter raises the issue of forces seemingly beyond our awareness or control, hostile forces from within and without that detract from processes that nurture human becoming. Chapter Five discusses a view of individuation set within the context of four powers helpful in sustaining human becoming. Chapter Six describes tapasya, the work of activating soul by taking the separative self and unfolding an awakening consciousness. Each chapter ends with practices designed to ground the theory, bring a living-force to the teachings, and open doorways to the inner journey. This text can be aligned with therapeutic processes as individuals access their own healthcare support system.

Part Two begins with Chapter Seven, which discusses the many and complex sides of subliminal consciousness, from personal to cosmic and universal. Chapter Eight focuses on Sri Aurobindo's complex notion of the emotional-vital being, raising challenging questions about consciousness and its formations and dynamic potential for destruction and reconstruction when Integral methods are adopted from a place of conscious awareness. Chapter Nine examines war-zone consciousness, the consciousness that sabotages upward intentions toward change and self-mastery. This state is discussed in terms of the involutionary and evolutionary process, and of a wide variety of personal and cosmic forces capable of detracting from positive motivational change. Chapter Ten outlines a multidimensional view of the mental biofield and the paradoxical development and use and misuse of thought forms. Chapter Eleven examines body consciousness from the physical and physical-etheric perspective, while Chapter Twelve expands on the role of subtle body consciousness by examining the body as the bridge and presenting ideas on how the unfolding of subtle consciousness impacts the physical, cellular, physiologic, and genetic substance of being. Chapter Thirteen presents Julia's Story (Julia is a pseudonym), a highly personal reflection presenting a tapasya of becoming.

Quotes from the clinical research settings are inter-spersed throughout the chapters in Part Two to reaffirm the unique and subjective nature of healing processes. (All names are pseudonyms.) Sri Aurobindo held that each person is unique and that while learning, growing, and claiming a life-path each individual can benefit from teachings and sustained support; however, in the end, each must seek inside for the true uniqueness of his or her purpose and dharma—service to humanity. Integrative Energy Healing within the context of this document is defined as: a subtle energy, intentional, full- spectrum therapeutic modality, that from within the context of awareness dialogue and specific biofield-based treatments, focuses on multidimensional physical, emotional, mental, and spiritual aspects of healing while clearing and restructuring the human subtle-body energy fields toward higher levels of coherence.

Part Three begins with Chapter Fourteen, which addresses a compilation of views that sustain sadhana as soul- work reiterating the complex interplay of Consciousness, Force, Energy, Light, and Information as it impacts the human condition. Included in this view are a range of ideas on rebirth and karma in Chapter Fifteen. Human becoming in Chapter Sixteen is framed under ideas that encourage and support lighting the flame of inquiry, placing the 'call' to spiritual practice and greater contribution within the context of inquiry. This chapter revisits the Gnostic transformational process and the three keys to change (aspiration, rejection, and surrender), as well as outlining the four powers in a manner that encourages further growth aimed at methods for reclaiming dharma. This chapter concludes with a summary of where we have been and where we can go in our human becoming as soul aspects are reclaimed and as consciousness is awakened to this great adventure.

The Epilogue, *Modern Day War Zone Consciousness*, examines some planetary challenges within the light of war zone consciousness as defined utilizing concepts from Integral yoga.

The text has been written to honor the wisdom of two great teachers, Sri Aurobindo and the Mother, Mira Alfassa, to show how wisdom can be timeless; moreover, how it can be applied at different times under different contexts: here our context is designed to empower individuals to develop transformative wellness based self-mastery skills that encompass the fullness of the human condition embracing both new science and the ancient world view of Consciousness, Force, Energy, Light, and Information, here meaning intuitive Knowledge or sophisticated multidimensional Information.

Part One:
Yoga of Self and Soul

1
Oneness and Consciousness

The master and Mover of our works is the One, the
Universal and Supreme, the Eternal and the Infinite...
the Self of all beings, the Master of all worlds,
transcending all worlds, the Light and the Guide,
the—Beautiful and All-Blissful, the Beloved and the
Lover...the Cosmic Spirit and all this creative Energy
around us...   - Sri Aurobindo (Ghose, 1996, p. 231).

We are One and also Relative—consciousness is
inherent in all existence. Each and all, animate and
inanimate, we are One. At the Absolute, we are One in
sachchidananda: Existence, Consciousness, and Bliss in
infinite arrays of form and force. But we are also Relative
and unique, whether animate or inanimate. The great
initiation for humankind is to learn the paradoxical yet
sacred practices bridging Absolute and Relative in ways
that develop the yoga of self and soul—with the ideal of
serving this beautiful planet and all humankind.

While views on consciousness are diverse and some
are highly materialistic, others bring interpretations that
sustain a new and holistic worldview. Especially in the West,
we say that everything is a materialistic phenomenon, but
is it? Is everything a material phenomenon capable of being
produced and interpreted by the brain and the senses? This
powerful, dominant worldview is fast becoming inadequate
in the face of the new Western science conjoined
with ancient Eastern teachings. New avenues for more
complex views of consciousness provide broader creative
perspectives that dramatically expand the possibilities of
human potential. Consistent with ancient Vedic teachings,
Sri Aurobindo removes the idea of consciousness in terms
of only mentality and indicates that consciousness is a self-

aware force inherent in all existence. It is, in essence, one and the same thing differently organized as a Force of Existence—a hidden intelligence. At its highest level, consciousness is *sachchidananda*: as *Sat*, it is pure pristine existence; as *Chit*, it is the energy that creates the worlds; as *Ananda*, it is bliss. At the highest supreme existence or state of Oneness (or Unity or Brahman in the Vedic teachings), consciousness is sachchidananda or Existence, Consciousness, Bliss. This state is not non-consciousness or non-existence, but is paradoxical and beyond words. It is a Nothingness that is a fullness of All, supreme beyond words and far beyond human cognitive understanding. Sri Aurobindo reminds us:

> Consciousness is a fundamental thing, the fundamental thing in existence—it is the energy, the motion, the movement of consciousness that creates the universe and all that is in it—not only the macrocosm but the microcosm is nothing but consciousness arranging itself.... Consciousness is a reality inherent in existence. It is there even when it is not active on the surface, but silent and immobile; it is there even when it is invisible on the surface, not reacting on outward things or sensible to them, but withdrawn and either active or inactive within; it is there even when it seems to us to be quite absent and the being to our view is unconscious and inanimate...there are ranges of consciousness above and below the human range, with which the normal human has no contact and they seem to be unconscious—[there are] supramental or overmental and submental ranges. (Ghose, 2000a, pp. 233-235).

Sri Aurobindo gathers all that is under the auspices of the immortal—so mortal we are, within the immortal, and understanding this truth of our being is the object of yoga. Ideas, principles, and all the forces and energies that exist are hollow moulds unless they imbibe of the transcendent Light of consciousness. This conscious

Oneness is present in all great spiritual traditions; in the Vedic tradition, Oneness can be termed Brahman and is Consciousness in its immortal inherent existence. Hence Oneness, Brahman, or the ultimate Reality (to others called God or Spirit) is much more than an abstract principle—it is a concrete experiential reality. Therefore, Consciousness is the Reality of all that is, luminous self- existence, reality at multi-levels. Consciousness is both self- revealing and dynamic, becoming all that is through complex hierarchical interweavings of Consciousness-Force.

Following years of inner experiential seeking, the ancient Rishis determined that Consciousness-Force works with three essential modes of Nature or *gunas*: *sattwa*, a force of equilibrium that brings peace, harmony and light; *rajas*, a force of kinesis that brings effort, struggle, passion, and action; and *tamas*, a force of inertia that brings incapacity, inaction, cohesion, and lack of motivation. These states are essentially aligned along a continuum and can be considered qualities of Nature that combine and underlie all movement (Ghose, 1996, 2000c).

More specifically, tamas as a principle brings inertia of force and of knowledge, leading to inaction, dull action, or mechanical, habitual, and nonreflective action: action easily propelled by outer forces. Tamas encourages ignorance, weakness, incapacity, cowardice, and a callous heart along with ignoble motives, conversely, it maintains stability.

The principle of rajas is intimately connected to the life force and the kinetic motor power but is driven by desire—it has to work against the inertia of tamas and therefore is characterized by effort and struggle. However, rajas has binding capacity and is needed at all times to some degree; it brings egoism, self-will, prejudice, pride and arrogance, selfish ambition, and vices and passions. Rajas also brings us the warrior and the men, women, and children who will speak for the wellbeing of humanity.

The principle of sattwa works closely with the mind,

intelligence, and reason, aiming to support the assimilation of knowledge, understanding, and will. Sattwa seeks mastery, light, and happiness; sattwa traits bring a balance of reason and ethics, clarity and disinterested truth, self-control, calmness, and a refined heart. However, Sri Aurobindo teaches that the most common guna is a combination of rajaso-tamasic, with desire habits and an impulsive nature (Ghose, 1996).

The yoga of self and soul works with the gunas, identifying how they and their forces play out in our lives. The ideal is a transformation of the gunas through spiritual purification processes, so that over time the sattwa guna becomes jyoti or clear spiritual light; rajas becomes tapas, a calm yet intense divine force; and tamas becomes sama, the divine stillness and peace. Sri Aurobindo explains how the force of the gunas influences the human condition and how transformative activities are needed if indeed the aim is a divinization, that is, a higher spiritual turn towards Oneness.

> In all things there is a presence, a primal Reality—the Self, the Divine, Brahman—which is forever pure, perfect, blissful, infinite: its infinity is not affected by the limitations of relative things; its purity is not stained by our sins and evil; its bliss is not touched by our pain and suffering; its perfection is not impaired by our defects of consciousness, knowledge, will, unity. (Ghose, 2000c, p. 409).

However, once we admit there is primal divine governance, we are left to concur that the governance is complete, unlimited, infinite, omnipresent, and omniscient. This governance also includes, then, the power and forces of darkness and evil steeped in Ignorance. Even for the human, this leaves existence as relative, freedom as relative. How are individuals solely responsible in this overall imperfection? To answer, it is necessary to find a place and significance for this division and suffering within the overall divine plan. What is the purpose of tamas, unruly rajas, and the veiled sattwa qualities of consciousness? Sri Aurobindo assures us that though life is a great mystery, there are conclusions to be drawn. He notes:

> The Divine Reality is infinite in its being; in this infinite being, we find limitations everywhere—that is the apparent fact from which our existence here seems to start and to which our own narrow ego and its ego-centric activities bear constant witness. But in reality, when we come to an integral self-knowledge, we find we are not limited, for we are also infinite. (Ghose, 2000c, p. 419).

Aurobindo assures us that no matter the degree of division, there is an overriding unity—division is the "surface results of an infinite multiplicity" (Ghose, 2000c, p. 419). There is imperfection and a divine will for humanity to transcend evil and suffering, and to transform imperfection in order to manifest a higher truth and meet with the ideal truth of being— in other words, to name the disguises of perfection. Sri Aurobindo assures:

> Our present nature can only be transitional, our imperfect status a starting-point and opportunity for the achievement of another higher, wider and greater that shall be divine and perfect not only by the secret spirit within it but in its manifest and most outward form of existence. (Ghose, 2000c, p. 414).

This mysterious and secret activity serves to provide the soul with guidance and a deeper understanding of the Ignorance. The adversity, stumbling, and pain bring teachings that support evolution toward a higher consciousness and greater understanding. The divine works out its intentions through the apparent ignorance—the teachings through struggle, pain, and suffering (or tapas) are designed to assist individuals to draw back from the surface state of being; to harmonize tamas, rajas, and sattwa; and to take actions that sustain their growing wisdom.

It is a fact of relative existence, a fact of world-consciousness, that humanity's limited forms of consciousness do cause grief, fear, anger, wars, dissonance, error, and falsehood in multiple ways and forms. It takes a deeper and wider consciousness to rise above the exact facts, values, and views of the moment to glean insight and aspire for different choices.

> ... every error is significant of the possibility and the effort of a discovery of truth; every weakness and failure is a first sounding of gulfs of power and potentiality; all division is intended to enrich by an experience of various sweetness of unification the joy of realised unity. All this imperfection is to us evil, but all evil is in travail of the eternal good; for all is an imperfection which is the first condition,... in the law of life evolving out of Inconscience,... of a greater perfection in the manifesting of the hidden divinity. But at the same time our present feeling of this evil and imperfection, the revolt of our consciousness against them is also a necessary valuation; for if we have first to face and endure them, the ultimate command on us is to reject, to overcome, to transform the life and the nature. It is for that end that their insistence is not allowed to slacken; the soul must learn the results of Ignorance, must begin to feel their reactions as a spur to its endeavour of mastery and conquest and finally to a greater endeavour of transformation and transcendence. (Ghose, 2000c, pp. 423-424).

At a deeper reality this is the law and these traits of Ignorance have their persistent reality.

While religions and philosophies differ as to the cause or Reality of this seeming paradox, Integral yoga offers a view of consciousness manifesting in infinite grades, each with its unique organization and purpose, setting steps for a progressive evolution of the soul or spiritual nature within each individual. Sri Aurobindo claims that at the level of divine Unity there must have been an ascent of the embodied spirit. He also says: "But it may be said that the reason for the Divine Will and delight in such a difficult and tormented progressive manifestation and the reason for the soul's assent to it is still a mystery" (Ghose, 2000c, p. 428). However, he does posit a perspective:

> ...a play of self-concealing and self-finding is one of the most strenuous joys that conscious being can give to itself, a play of extreme attractiveness. There is no greater pleasure...than a victory in creation over the impossibilities of creation, a delight in the conquest over an anguished toil and a hard ordeal of suffering. At the end of separation is the intense joy of union, the joy of meeting with a self from which we were divided. (Ghose, 2000c, p. 428).

The meta-process includes three steps: realization of the individual, then a higher order universal, and finally the transcendent merging with Oneness while still maintaining individuality within the Oneness. Called tapasya, this intense work brings a multi-dynamic play of consciousness with the qualities of tamas, rajas, and sattwa as they interpenetrate each of the aspects of consciousness. When the work is done on behalf of this special toil, the toil unfolds consciousness on behalf of the One, in answer to an unnameable longing deep in the centre of our being.

To understand the metaphysics behind such a stance it is useful to understand how Sri Aurobindo articulates the role of Consciousness as an involution and evolution of Consciousness- Force.

INTEGRAL REFLECTION PRACTICES

Throughout time, individuals have written about distinct experiences of the individual, universal, and transcendent.

Your view:

1. Take time to truly come into your own being, to your own personal individuality. Who are you? Ask, "Who am I?" Spend time with this question, and journal your thoughts from at least three different perspectives.

2. Recall a time when you felt the 'universal'. It could have been stimulated by a starry night sky, a beautiful piece of music, or the smile of a loved one. How did this feel? Find three different perspectives.

3. Have you experienced a sense of the transcendent? If you have, what was this like for you? If you have not, what might this be like for you? Journal your impressions.

2
Separation: Involution and Evolution

... the seat of the Transcendent Consciousness is above in an absoluteness of divine Existence—and there too is the absolute Power, Truth, Bliss of the Eternal—of which our mentality can form no conception and of which even our greatest spiritual experience is only a diminished reflection in the spiritualised mind and heart, a faint shadow, a thin derivative.

Yet proceeding from there is a sort of golden corona of Light, Power, Bliss and Truth—a divine Truth- Consciousness as the ancient mystics called it, a Supermind, a Gnosis, with which this world of a lesser consciousness proceeding by Ignorance is in secret relation and which alone maintains and prevents it from falling into a disintegrating chaos... there lie many levels of ascending consciousness, highest mental or overmental, which we would have to conquer before we arrived there or could bring down its greatest glory here.

Yet however difficult that ascent, that victory is the destiny of the human spirit and that luminous descent of bringing down of that divine Truth is the inevitable term of the troubled evolution of the earth-nature; the intended consummation is its raison d'etre, our culminating state and the explanation for our terrestrial existence.

– Sri Aurobindo (Ghose, 1996, p. 242).

Consciousness-Force is described as a twofold movement: involution and evolution. *Involution* in this context means that all is silent, formless, and self-contained: "Consciousness seems to be involved in an obscure nothingness, an abyss of blind Force forever engrossed in its own dark whirl" (Satprem, see Enginger, 1993, p. 253). With involution, all is contained in the seed. Satprem continues, "Without this involution no evolution would be possible, for how could something come out of nothing?" (p. 254). For evolution to occur, individuals must grasp the fire of the soul, "the leader of the journey and the key, the secret evolutionary impetus" (p. 255). What is this evolutionary impetus? In this chapter we examine the broad and complex view of involution and evolution and their impact on the organization of human consciousness.

At one end of the spectrum, Consciousness-Force is static and immovable, All-Knowing, and evolved; at the other, Ignorance is inconscient, forgetting, and involved. Nevertheless, Sri Aurobindo (Ghose, 2000a, 2000b) reassures us that though deeply involved, the All-Knowing is present but far removed by the separative movement of Tapas. He likens Consciousness- Force to a reservoir that the water channels use when required, without being aware of it—as if there is a sea somewhere, resting in a deep state.

This great sea of Consciousness-Force is aware of the past, present, and future. While living in three times, it is aware of the infinite potentialities of existence; moreover, the three times are "present all the time at the back of the consciousness and in the work itself" and influence how potentialities unfold (Ghose, 2000a, p. 610). Sri Aurobindo states that Consciousness- Force living in three times is one rationale for *karma*, the link between the past and its effect on the future. For humans, the involved Consciousness-Force is aware of the smallest memory- based aspect of the past, while humans themselves only remember a conceptual, ghostly aspect of the past.

Sri Aurobindo (Ghose, 2000a) argues that from a cosmic perspective Ignorance has truth and a role in the involution- evolution process. There is, he insists, a spiritual economy and an assigned place for Ignorance. Without it, all we experience could be considered an "unreal creation of the Absolute, [such that] both cosmic and individual existence would be in their very nature an Ignorance; the sole real knowledge would be the indeterminable self-awareness of the Absolute" (p. 336). Thus, all cosmic and individual existence is placed within the context of a spiritual Reality in the process of becoming; Ignorance is a subordinate power necessary for this purpose to unfold in time.

Guided by the nature and will of Tapas, Consciousness-Force spans the full continuum from complete Absolute awareness to apparent absolute inconscience. Infinite spans of Consciousness-Force work within what Sri Aurobindo terms the Energy of nature, an Energy directed by Tapas or Will (Ghose, 1996, 2000a).

Guided by Consciousness-Force and Tapas, the involution–evolutionary process leads to planes of being, consciousness, and existence. These planes are formed through a subtle continuity of levels of Consciousness-Force involving into forgetfulness and conversely evolving back to awakened awareness (Ghose, 1996, 2000a).

Sri Aurobindo outlines two systems that assist the understanding of this complex play of existence. He speaks of the *horizontal concentric system* of organization as containing parts of the being, with superimposed layers of consciousness constituting the *hierarchical system*. There are three circles in the horizontal concentric system: outer being, inner being, and innermost being. Conversely, the hierarchical system is based on a ladder-like escalation of consciousness. (Ghose, 1996, 2000a).

The concentric model shown below separates (a) the outer or surface aspects of the being that are usually congealed into an amorphous, prerational or egoic-rational personality- state, from (b) those aspects of inner being that are immersed in the subliminal, and (c) the innermost soul consciousness—true being.

Dalal (2007a) describes this system as follows:

The concentric system is like a series of rings or sheaths, consisting of the outer being, the inner being and the inmost being. The outer being and the inner being behind it constitute our phenomenal or instrumental being and are said to belong to Nature....They have three corresponding parts—physical, vital, mental. The inmost being is the... true being (p. 201).

The *outer being* consists of the mental being, the vital or life-force (or emotional being, as it is called), and the physical body-consciousness. Each of the outer and inner beings has its own consciousnesses, and more than one type of conscious awareness is present in each area. *Mind* refers to mental cognition, ideas, and thoughts—all part of intelligent actions. The *vital* or emotional is based on desire, sensations, feelings, passions, and a whole array of emotions including anger, jealousy, envy, fear, greed, excitement, pleasure, and so on. The vital is full of impulses and life-force pushes to fulfill desire- based needs; it is fixed on movement and drama, whether induced by or inducing pain or pleasure. The body, while appearing to run on mainly mechanical impulse, is itself a conscious organism with the ability to obey all natural healthy impulses from inside and outside, or to rebel following the whim of the vital, the mental, or its own unknown inner impulsions (Dalal, 2001; Vrinte, 2002). This body-consciousness is mainly unknown by the surface mind.

The *inner being* (or subliminal being), a far larger aspect of our being, is concealed under the surface—hidden behind the veil of ordinary life, behind the outer being vital, mind, and body. Below, beneath, behind, and above ordinary consciousness, as complex as that consciousness is in itself, lies an amazing world of subtle consciousness and awareness capable of linking all aspects of being into oneness. Universal Consciousness-Force can access the inner mind, inner vital, and inner or subtle physical. Sri Aurobindo (Ghose, 2000a, 2000c) speaks of the subtle

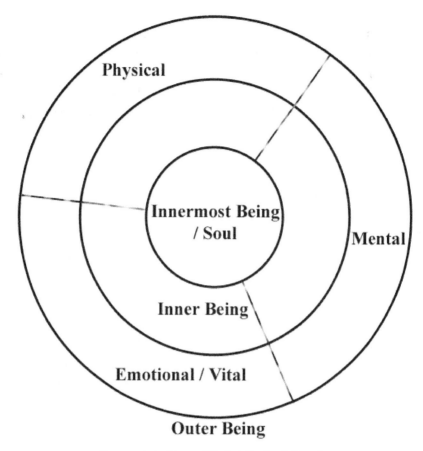

Concentric Map with Subliminal Overlay

consciousness and subliminal consciousness of the inner mind, inner vital, and subtle physical systems— systems that have access to a greater understanding of self and life.

The evolutionary development process is designed to access the wisdom of these hidden realms. Dalal (2007a) clarifies:

> Behind the surface or frontal consciousness of the outer being there is an inner or subliminal consciousness upon all the three levels—physical, vital, mental. Thus there is an inner mind, an inner vital and an inner physical. The inner mind is in touch with the universal mind, the inner vital with universal life-forces, and the inner physical with the

universal physical forces around us. Thus where the outer being knows things only indirectly from their outer touches as perceived through the senses and the outer mind, the inner being is directly aware of the surrounding universal forces that act through us (p. 203).

And Sri Aurobindo (Ghose, 2000c) reminds us that "the inner being—inner mind, inner vital, inner or subtle physical— knows much that is unknown to the outer mind, the outer vital, the outer physical, for it is direct contact with the secret forces of Nature" (p. 269). It is "the inner being—inner mind, inner vital, inner or subtle physical" (p. 269) that warns us and gives us intimations about our actions.

Another aspect of the subliminal consciousness, the *innermost being* is the psychic being or soul consciousness—a spark of the eternal, a portion of the Divine. It develops through many lifetimes, organizing the inner and outer being around its own essence and presence. The psychic being does not die with the body but leaves, goes to supraphysical planes of existence between earthly incarnations, and after a period of assimilation and rest, selects and enters a new body near the time of rebirth. The psychic being remains behind the veil of the outer personality and its activity, influencing and indirectly guiding the surface life until a certain level of development and self-mastery has been achieved.

The psychic being, or *chaitya purusha* (popularly referred to as the soul) is directly connected with the transcendent sachchidananda; as Pandit (1983) so beautifully reminds us, "it is always the fresh radiance, a divine ray" (p. 23). He elucidates:

> But in most it is hidden, concealed, overlaid by veils, layers after layers of ignorance, emotional crusts. As the individual grows in evolution, as he refines himself, gets over the murk of desires,

passions, anger, hatred and things that are dark, as
he refines through culture, ethics, devotion, self-
sacrifice, self-giving, the crust thins, the veils tear...
then the passage is cleared and the psychic action
takes place more and more frequently (p. 23-24).
Sri Aurobindo inspires with certitude:

At a certain stage in the Yoga when the mind is
sufficiently quieted and no longer supports itself
at every step on the sufficiency of its mental
certitudes, when the vital has steadied and subdued
and is no longer constantly insistent on its own
rash will, demand and desire, when the physical has
sufficiently altered not to bury altogether the inner
flame under the mass of its outwardness, obscurity
or inertia, an inmost being hidden within and felt
only in its rare influences is able to come forward
and illumine the rest and take up the lead of the
Sadhana....it has in it a flame of will insistent on
perfection, on an alchemic transmutation of all the
inner and outer existence. (Ghose, 1996, pp. 145-
146).

This innermost being, the psychic being is the part
from which one can most easily access the Spirit. Sri
Aurobindo makes great effort to ensure seekers are guided
clearly, describing the soul's awareness:

In the first long stage of its growth and immature
existence it has leaned on earthy love, affection,
tenderness, goodwill, compassion, benevolence, on
all beauty and gentleness and fineness and light and
strength and courage, on all that can help to refine
and purify the grossness and commonness of human
nature; but it knows how mixed are these human
movements at their best and at their worst how
fallen and stamped with the mark of ego and self-
deceptive sentimental falsehood and the lower
self profiting by the imitation of a soul movement.
(Ghose, 1996, p. 146).

Dalal (2011) notes that it is the evolution of soul consciousness in the psychic being that determines our inner personality and brings forth the outer circumstances in our lives.

Integral to this yoga are depth teachings about moving below the surface, diving deeply into a silent, immobile sweetness where time is eternal and the core of the soul reveals itself. When fully achieved, Sri Aurobindo (1996, 2000a, 2000c) calls this the *psychicisation* of the being, a process that encompasses reaching a dynamic place of positive peace and wisdom that guides with surety.

The soul or psychic being and the inner mental, inner vital, and subtle physical—all aspects of the subliminal consciousness—connect to each other and to the outer mental, vital, physical consciousness and the outer world. The inner and innermost aspects of our being are part of the multifaceted subliminal consciousness (Ghose, 1996, 2000a), a consciousness filled with esoteric wisdom that rests dynamically and statically behind the outer awareness. This inner plane is larger, wider, and more luminous in consciousness than the outer surface consciousness; the innermost plane stands behind and is interwoven with the inner mental, inner vital, and subtle physical. The subliminal consists of a luminously informed and efficient mind, a powerful vital, and a subtle, fluid physical, bringing involutionary and evolutionary processes together and providing amazing abilities for intercommunication among all the planes of being.

The subliminal consciousness is connected to the outer planes and personality through centers of consciousness called *chakras*. Sri Aurobindo says that "only a little of the inner being escapes through these centers into the outer life, but that is the best part of ourselves" (as quoted by Dalal, 2007b, p. 350).

There are seven major chakras situated in and along the spine, each with a Sanskrit name, each carrying a different type of multidimensional consciousness combined with hundreds of minor chakras situated at nerve plexus and bone articulation sites throughout the body. Sri Aurobindo divides the chakras into three sets as follows.

1. The physical chakras: the first chakra (the Muladahara chakra) governing physical consciousness and the subconscient;

2. The vital being chakras: the second chakra (the Swadhisthana) governing lower vital movements; the third chakra (the Manipura) governing larger vital forces, passions, and desires; and the fourth chakra (the Anahata) that holds the outer desire nature and the inner soul access;

3. The mental chakras: the fifth chakra (the Visuddha) governing the physical mind and outer physical things; the sixth chakra (the Ajna) governing the dynamic mind, thought, vision, and inner will opening to yogic consciousness; and the seventh chakra (the Sahasrara) governing the superconscient planes of higher mind to Sachchidananda (Dalal, 2007b).

The developing chakras create the *auric field*, or levels of the human energy field—in essence, these layers of the field are dynamic representations of energy and consciousness in the physical, emotional-vital, mental, and spiritual aspects of ourselves. These layers interpenetrate throughout our being: from atom to molecule, cell, and tissue, and from physical matter to the inner being's increasingly subtle aspects of our presentation as an individual. These subtle layers also dynamically interact with our environment or *circumconscient field*. Hence, the inner being and outer being are radically and dynamically interconnected with each other and the environment.

The subliminal consciousness has access to the nonlocal realms, realms that transcend space and time. This consciousness performs a psychospiritual function: It opens individuals through these centers to the subtle nonmaterial organs of perception often termed high-sense perception or extended perception. Additionally, supraphysical and subconscient planes of consciousness are accessible when these centers are sufficiently open (Ghose, 1996, 2000a; Dalal, 2007a).

The environmental consciousness (or circum-conscient) is a formulation of the subliminal consciousness projecting itself deeply into and beyond the physical body. This consciousness in humans, often called the aura, receives waves of universal force and picks up thoughts, feelings, and sensations from the surrounding environment and beyond. For example, strong desire thought-forms can impact the auric field; in other words, mind waves, emotional-vital waves, feeling, and sensation waves can all enter a vulnerable auric field, and if not identified as foreign aspects of consciousness, can impact the individual's thought, feeling, and action (Dalal, 2007a).

All consciousness has an environmental field—the more consciousness is set and formulated, the greater the environmental field. Fields with the most force and dynamic power impact the surrounding environment more than diffuse and unfocused waves of Consciousness-Force and Tapas.

Involution and evolution on the personality and egoic level relate intimately with Sri Aurobindo's view of consciousness. The discussion now turns to the hierarchical model that overlays and lies beneath the concentric view. Here Sri Aurobindo adds another aspect to his highly enriching view of existence.

In this model shown below, the hierarchical, vertical planes of being transcend from low to high vibrational status as follows: the inconscient, subconscient, physical, vital, mental, higher mind, illumined mind, intuitive mind, overmind, supermind, and sachchidananda which dissolves into Brahman, or pure Reality (Dalal, 2001). The inconscient is the nethermost aspect of consciousness, the place of the deepest sleep, and the place of the most misguided Tapas—this is the place of maximum involution

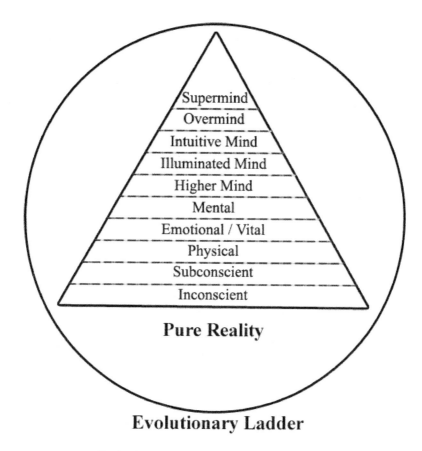

Evolutionary Ladder

Evolutionary Ladder within Pure Reality

of consciousness where the struggle to evolve is at its most resistive.

Sri Aurobindo describes the *inconscience* as "an inverse reproduction of the supreme superconscience: it has the same absoluteness of being and automatic action, but in a vast involved trance; it is lost in itself, plunged in its own abyss of infinity... darkness veiled within darkness" (Dalal, 2001, p. 349). Above the total involution of consciousness of the inconscient lies the subconscient, near the physical consciousness. The subconscient is an obscure consciousness that passively receives into itself impressions from the mental, vital, and physical consciousness immersed in desires, sensations, nervous reactions, mechanistic patterns, physical habits, fixed notions, mechanical thoughts, obstinate tendencies, dreams, and samskaras (habitual impulsions). According to Sri Aurobindo, this consciousness is "largely responsible for our illnesses; chronic or repeated illnesses are indeed mainly due to the subconscient and its obstinate memory and habit of repetition of whatever has impressed itself upon the body-consciousness" (as quoted by Dalal, 2001, p. 350).

The subconscient holds onto impressions and usurps the rational thinking processes by sending these impressions to the surface just as change could occur; it holds onto the repetition of complexes, wounding, and sorrows, obstinately refusing transformation. Sri Aurobindo notes:

> The subconscient is the main cause why all things repeat themselves and nothing ever gets changed except in appearance. It is the cause why people say character cannot be changed, the cause also of the constant return of things one hoped to have got rid of forever. (Dalal, 2001, p. 350).

This level of obscure consciousness is known to strongly influence the outer, waking consciousness as well as much of the dream state.

The subconscient is also an entrance for Ignorance, where untoward ideas and thoughts can enter, controlling the individual like a slave. It is also here that hostile vital beings (subtle energetic forms from the etheric or astral planes) can enter, stay, and possess individuals (Ghose & Alfassa, 2004; Reddy, 2007).

> Importantly, Sri Aurobindo and the Mother observed that hostile vital beings are polymorphic in nature and can manifest themselves in various forms, according to mental scheme of different times and cultures. Thus, the demons and devils of old ... are related phenomena that involve the same hostile forces that have been plaguing humanity since its beginning. (Miovic, 2007, p. 44).

Also included in the hierarchical model are the characteristics of the outer and inner aspects of the physical, vital, and mental consciousness, which were outlined above in the description of the concentric model of consciousness. From the hierarchical perspective, the vibrational Consciousness-Force and Tapas are distinct from the subconscient and encompass numerous higher levels of consciousness above the ordinary human mind. Higher mind is the next vibrational aspect above the rational mind and the first plane of spiritual consciousness. This consciousness has a higher, nonlogic-based thought-power, a spiritual character, and a broader and wider view; it presents ideas to the mind in a clear and accessible manner once the mind itself has been prepared and purified in readiness to receive (Dalal, 2007a; Ghose, 2000a, 2000b).

Illumined mind is a higher and purer domain of consciousness that holds what Sri Aurobindo calls spiritual light, as well as a larger, wiser, and vaster spiritual-conceptual awareness. The illumined mind brings peace and yet can descend into our being with force, power, and drive, Truth-Sight, or direct 'Knowing' reaching beyond higher mind to spiritual light provides for a calm, peaceful, and vast descent of knowledge into our daily awareness (Dalal, 2007a; Ghose, 2000a).

The intuitive level characterized in this hierarchical model is not to be confused with ordinary aspects of intuition; rather, the intuition referred to here is close to knowledge by identity. This intuitive level brings a truth-perception, a complete identification with wisdom and awareness so strong that certainty of correctness is unquestionable (though still to be reflected upon to ascertain that the lower mind has not interwoven its own ideas). This intuitional plane is one that encompasses inspiration, revelation, and swift discrimination; it is a consciousness of Truth-flashes, Truth-perception, Truth- ideas, and direct vision (Dalal, 2001; Ghose, 2000a).

Overmind is the division point whereby the duality of mind meets with the indivisible knowledge of supermind; it supports the present evolutionary status of individuals while remaining full of light and power. Overmind consciousness is expansive, beyond time and space, and globally aware; it is the plane of Gods, Goddesses, and cosmic conscious perception (Dalal, 2001; Ghose, 2000a).

Above the overmind consciousness lies the supermind, and as Dalal (2001) comments, this is a "radically different" (p.356) consciousness—it is Truth-Consciousness. As Sri Aurobindo explained:

> The Supermind is in its very essence a truth-consciousness, a consciousness always free from the Ignorance which is the foundation of our present natural or evolutionary existence and from which nature in us is trying to arrive at self-knowledge and world-knowledge and a right consciousness and the right use of our existence in the universe..... its very nature is knowledge: it has not to acquire knowledge but possesses it in its own right.... (as quoted by Dalal, 2001, p. 356).

Importantly, supermind is the intermediary between the One and the Many, or the Absolute Reality and all separate being—it is the creative consciousness that brings the many into manifestation out of unity consciousness. This consciousness holds both the one and the many simultaneously within itself, and so holds the many together and in relation with the one. It supports the evolution of consciousness leading to the highest bliss and a fully soul-based, spiritualised, and universalized world-consciousness.

Last in this hierarchy is the triune sachchidananda, the supracosmic reality—the Existence, Consciousness, and Bliss of harmony in multiplicity. This One and timeless eternal existence is Transcendent, Self-aware, self-blissful, pure, conscious infinite Existence.

The foundations for the yoga of self and soul are set within the context of Oneness at the Absolute, and within the involutionary and evolutionary movement of consciousness at the relative. Each step in the conscious evolutionary process is a tapasya, a work of the soul that occurs in stages inherent to the teachings of Integral yoga.

In the next chapters a three-stage process is interwoven with main practices that bring life to the theory: first, centralizing the ego and understanding and healing the fractured ego; second, unfolding the soul, or individualization; and third, psychicising or soul activation. Each stage takes the theory of Integral yoga to a new level of complexity and experiential practice: Each understanding and practice is designed to activate conscious awareness in a gentle yet poignantly refreshing and creative manner.

INTEGRAL REFLECTION PRACTICES

We come with freedom and choice as part of our karmic conditioning, a part of our self-heritage. When we are not in 'awakening choice' we are in habit, and habitual mind takes over with its array of conditioned responses. Our task, or tapasaya (work of the soul) is to develop discernment skill— the skills for 'being conscious'. This type of discernment requires a precise application of force in order to unfold the consciousness that brings 'self-awareness' to the foreground.

*1. **Notice what you notice**. This practice requires that you become aware that you are aware—you develop 'lucid conscious noticing'.*

Process: Select set times in the day in which you agree to develop extraordinary sense awareness. Begin with short spans of time, even two or three minutes, and later extend these times. Discern among the outer being physical, emotional-vital, and mental reactions/responses to life experience. Identify environmental (circumconscient) influences on your outer being physical, emotional-vital, and mental reactions/ responses. Journal these impressions.

*2. **Name conditioned-self reactions**. The majority of our reactions are subconscious habits; the work of evolution is the practice of becoming conscious.*

Process: Notice your conditioned reactions, particularly the ones that cause strife in your life.

In an open, curious, and nonjudgmental manner, notice each aspect of the reaction. Bring to awareness the causative trajectory, or your initial ideas on how this reaction formed and why.

Reflect on a more positive and productive response. Then slowly begin to release this habit pattern and replace it with a positive response. Note with care and attention how you do this and how you feel physically, emotionally, mentally, and spiritually as you reformulate a new response. Journal this process on a few targeted conditioned-self reactions that you wish to change.

3
Centralising: Developing the Ego

The formulation of a mental and vital ego tied to the body-sense was the first great labour of the cosmic Life in its progressive evolution; for this was the means it found for creating out of matter a conscious individual.

-Sri Aurobindo (Ghose, 1996, p. 341).

Consciousness-Force and Tapas are active in human development, with the nature of Tapas leading consciousness into and out of the involved state necessary for human development. Sri Aurobindo tells us: "The present actor, poet, or soldier in himself is only a separative determination of Tapas; it is his force of being organized for a particular kind of action of its energy" (Ghose, 2000a, p. 609). In other words, mind and matter are different grades of consciousness, which is also Energy. In this thinking the brain is not the originator- consciousness; rather, consciousness uses the brain and is active in various degrees of awareness in all of its infinite ways of manifesting. In this chapter, I discuss how consciousness manifests and contributes to ego development from the perspective of the concentric model (Dalal, 2000).

The yoga of awakening to the self and soul process has many facets, among which developing the ego is primary. As this awareness presents in the outer and inner being concentric model, a view through the lens of Consciousness-Force and Tapas provides a construct from which to discuss a sophisticated yogic view of the ego.

Humans are immersed in a great cosmic play. Initially born into the pre-egoic state, emerging out of a primordial unconsciousness and bliss, a person has the opportunity to develop a *conscious ego*—a separate and independent, centralized sense of self. Without this, Sri Aurobindo states, the person remains a more-or-less amorphous entity, fused with others and the environment. Dalal (2000) speaks of the necessity for each individual to become individualized, to develop a conscious egoic state of being. Developing ego is a key in this process; even if this development is immersed in the outer superficial, it still serves to lift the person out of the unconscious.

Ego development is a progressive process that for most people remains, as Sri Aurobindo comments, a half-conscious and half-unconscious existence—a partial egoic state and partial pre- egoic state, and for some perhaps a post-egoic or individuated state (Ghose, 2000a). Success brings forth a new dimension of evolution: "Once the separative ego has been adequately developed evolution of consciousness can be accelerated through growth in a different dimension" (Dalal, 2000, p. v).

Sri Aurobindo discusses a Beyond ego or individualized state; however, before traversing Beyond ego, cautions in the literature encourage an initial, full, and secure development of ego. Vannucci (2005), discussing psychoanalysis framed by Integral yoga, advocates the development of a consistent, wide, and flexible egoic-personality base, describing the necessity to have "...a strong body and strong nerves... you must have a strong basis of equanimity in your external being" (p. 19). She reiterates that this equanimity must sustain an ego sturdy enough to address the deeply ingrained fears present since childhood (or even from previous incarnations), as such fears bring much trauma and are the cause, in her view, of the majority of illnesses.

The concentric model with its outer physical, emotional- vital, and mental forces of consciousness explains the most prevalent and empowered aspect of our nature after birth. Tapasya, developing higher, broader, and deeper powers of awareness—unfolding consciousness— requires the ability to become more aware of consciousness and all its different degrees and powers. These degrees include the multiple dimensional physical, emotional-vital, mental, and spiritual of both the outer and inner being.

To start, let's examine the outer being, the outermost ring of the concentric model emphasizing the key role of the mind as guardian of clarity, understanding, and discernment, and as a keeper of wisdom. The physical body is often *tamasic* (slow to change) and mechanical in its functioning, yet Sri Aurobindo tells us that the body is secretly conscious and capable of responding to both the emotional-vital and mental state of our being. The body can manifest within its cells and tissues the commands— conscious or unconscious—of the vital and the mind (and, in certain cases, even from the environment.) Conversely, the body itself impacts vital and mental states of being. This physical consciousness or body-consciousness has both surface and subcontient features, and of course, is impacted by the innermost soul nature. However, its main traits link with tamas, habit, and mechanical patterned activities.

The emotional-vital, enamored of change and intimately rajasic, is largely submerged in the subconscient; it aims to control the rest of the being and is characteristically easily distracted from both inside and outside. The vital likes a dispersion of consciousness and scattered perspectives— conflict, agitation, and emotional extremes seem to feed it. Duality, with its pairs of opposites, creates a constant disequilibrium; excitement and disquiet are frequent visitors. Maintaining separateness and independence is a constant preoccupation.

Development of the egoic consciousness relies on the emotional-vital becoming conscious, distinguishable from body- sensation, so that a sense-mind and intelligence can form. In essence, there are three aspects to the emotional-vital. First is a mental or higher-vital that allows emotions and feelings, passions and desires to be articulated; the higher-vital is often the home of creative ideas and visions, and when purified, provides a link with the soul. Second is an emotional-vital that is the seat of feelings such as love, joy, sorrow, and grief, and the home of stronger reactions and impulsions such as fear, greed, and more egoistic ambitions. Last, the physical-vital is closely aligned to the nervous system and the physiological needs, desires, and sensations of the body.

There can be no unity or wholeness when the emotional-vital reigns, and the template for emotional-vital reactiveness is formulated in the early years. Sri Auroboindo says: "Most people live in the vital. That means that they live in their desires, sensations, emotional feelings, vital imaginations, and see and experience everything from this point of view" (Ghose, 2000, p. 1297).

The mind also formulates itself early in life as traits develop. Sri Aurobindo explains that one common view is the rajaso-tamasic, in which individuals become stuck in narrow ideas or passionately rigid worldviews. As other traits take leadership through human development, the mind can become more sattwic and balanced in its views by seeking knowledge and using reason, learning how to problem solve, and integrating values. Strengthening and aligning Consciousness-Force and Tapas is required for egoic development and for ego surpassing.

As with the physical and emotional-vital being, both inner and outer, there are multiple grades or subplanes of mind consciousness. Humans often function simultaneously on numerous of these planes—this discussion focuses on the *physical-mind*, *emotional-vital-mind*, *thought-mind*, and *spiritual-mind*.

The physical-mind depends on the physical brain for facts and feedback from the five senses. Objective observance and external views are prominent here.

In Integral yoga the mind specifically has a large role; however, as can be seen, it is not the whole of consciousness as defined in the ordinary use of the term. In this yoga we learn to separate the outer and inner aspects, using a witness view and differentiating mind from the emotional-vital and body consciousness. For example, the body consciousness is more nervous and sensational as well as automatic, and this gradation of awareness differs from mind.

The body has its own sensate feeling—often before the mind has registered an event. The physical-mind is skeptical of the supraphysical, and even after a spiritual experience will forget it quickly. And the vital is highly responsive, desire ridden and capable of overwhelming the sattwic mental calm. The vital mind keeps us in set worldviews, easily disallowing new or broader perspectives.

> The vital mind...perceives the actual, the physical, the objective and accepts it as fact and this fact as self- evident truth beyond question; whatever is not actual, not physical, not objective it regards as unreal or unrealized, only to be accepted as entirely real when it has succeeded in becoming actual, becoming a physical fact, becoming objective... (Sri Aurobindo, as cited by Dalal, 2001, p. 54).

The physical-mind is the first mental status to evolve, and early in life its habitual and mechanical nature is supportive of human development.

Above this mind lies a more dynamic emotional-vital-mind whereby the vital intentions can enslave the mental faculties to obtain desires and ambitions from an egoic perspective. Conversely, the vital-dominated individual can also use the higher-vital to introduce new ideas, break up the status quo, champion worthy causes, and open the way for new evolutionary forces. The vital mind holds dreams, visions, and the imagination that births unique ideas. It is highly subjective and imaginative, and seeks emotive satisfaction.

Rajasic, this mind disturbs the tamasic physical-mind's external-driven sensate consciousness. Rajasically also, it demands more and more: more possibilities, new worlds to conquer. Individuals who successfully take leadership positions have an active vital-mind, as may those who fantasize great adventures. Much of the vital-mind is egoic-based and designed to satisfy a will or desire for power or possession. Additionally, if the next mental sublevel is active, much can be accomplished

Above the vital-mind subplane is the thought-mind, which brings a depth of thought and intelligence that may or may not dominate the person. When activated, this subplane creates the scientist, philosopher, seer, visionary dreamer, poet, and creator of ideas. Here, discriminating reason, intuitions, and direct insight contribute to judgment—again it depends which is stronger, the vital push to the mental or the thinking to support the mental consciousness.

Once the reflective aspects prevail, the pure thinker inside is empowered, though there is still a veil between the thought-mind and knowledge of the Truth. Depending on the individual's clarity, degrees of truth prevail. The mental "...gets the real truth only when something else puts a higher light into it..." (Ghose, 2000b, p. 1247). This more evolved mind-state is capable of carefully observing facts and processes, reasoning and making deductions, changing perspectives, and when the witness noticing state is active, changing worldviews when observations and intuitions determine that the time for change has arrived. Then individuals can determine what their nature is used to and habituated to, versus the higher sense of a truth unfolding; or conversely, they can grasp that they are impacted by waves and currents of mental energy entering from outside, contrary to what they feel is true internally.

The spiritual-mind subplane brings an impulse for truth-seeking and a power, though often veiled, for truth-finding. Sri Aurobindo tells us that those with a developed higher mental faculty cannot transform their nature, but they can impact and harmonize it by imposing rules, sublimating and refining it, and bringing insight and understanding to the "confusion and conflict or the summary patchwork of our divided and half-constructed being" (Ghose, 2000c, pp. 717-720; see also Dalal, 2001, p. 46). Individuals accessing this plane can consciously contribute to self-creation and truth-formation. The next step in Integral yoga is spiritual development integrated with the unfolding of higher aspects of mind, accompanied by access to the inner and innermost being.

However, in the development of the ego—the centralized and functional self of daily life—the outer physical, emotional, and mental aspects of being are necessary. Indeed, in Integral yoga they are necessary in a more profound manner than is customary. It is important to initially discern the three large outer-being formulations of consciousness and then slowly and diligently, with patience, understanding, discrimination, and kindness, name the subplane configurations of consciousness as they enhance or detract from ego development.

The Mother herself asks: "Unless you know who you are, and have a true sense of your own individuality, how can you give yourself to anything or anyone?" (Alfassa, 2005). Hence, this centralizing, egoic-personality structure is a principle worthy of consideration within the context of yogic development.

With a mature healthy ego, the individual can withstand the inner examination and purification required to heal the fractured egoic aspects and to soften ego resistance, admitting spiritualised consciousness. This softened and healthy ego is more consciously open to the deep underlying Consciousness- Force. Then, "misapplication of knowledge, miscombination, misconstruction, misrepresentation, a complicated machinery of mental error" can be, if not avoided, at least reduced (Ghose, 2000a, pp. 642-643). The inner and innermost concentric processes are elaborated on in Part Two, where we explore the fracturing of the ego more completely, a process requiring much more awareness of both the concentric and hierarchical interconnections.

The ego is known to veil the Divine and the subliminal and subtle inner physical, emotional-vital, and mental being; however, as the ego develops, centralizes, and softens, it becomes more porous, receives higher wisdom, and can access higher principles of being. The evolutionary push for ego transcendence gains force. Nevertheless, with a gaining of overall force of consciousness, the vital aspects and tamasic- rajasic forces keen to prevail in the consciousness bring innumerable challenges. It is important to stabilize each step by utilizing practices that support and sustain the evolution of consciousness.

INTEGRAL REFLECTION PRACTICES

Our ego helps us formulate ourselves; it gives us a basis for moving inward to assess thoughts, feelings, sensations, and spiritual motives, as well as moving outward to perceive the external world. Ego attaches us to the self of habit and conditionality, gives us a sense of 'noticing', and initiates boundaries.

1. Witnessing: Notice what you are feeling, sensing, and thinking at this moment. Take each attribute and journal a description. Discern aspects of feeling, body-sensing, and thinking.

2. Refocusing: Can you differentiate again, even more clearly? Journal this perspective.

3. From this point are you able to 'notice that you notice' differences?

4. Take this exercise farther and see if you can differentiate your physical, emotional, mental, and spiritual boundaries in an instance of your choice during your busy day.

5. Can you name what, for you, an unhealthy 'noticing' might be? A healthy 'noticing'? A strategy for changing an unhealthy 'noticing' to a healthy noticing? This practice further develops 'witness' consciousness.

6. Once you are able to differentiate among the outer physical, emotional-vital, and mental plane configurations of consciousness during normal daily activities, focus more on your 'reactive' moments when these habitual reactions no longer serve the growth of a healthy ego. Initiate new, healthy egoic response patterns. Journal examples of this process.

7. Spend time in gratitude and honor your process while steadfastly working toward your ideal.

4
Dissolution: Fracturing the Ego

In the cosmos, there are higher forces of the Divine
Nature—forces of Light, Truth, divine Power, Peace,
Ananda—there are the forces of the lower nature
which belong either to a lower truth or to ignorance
and error— there are also hostile forces whose whole
aim is to maintain the reign of Darkness, falsehood,
Death and Suffering as the law of life.
-Sri Aurobindo (Ghose, 1996, p. 142).

The hostile forces are there in the world to maintain
the Ignorance...because they [have] the right to
test the sincerity of the sadhaks [seekers] in their
power and will to cleave to the Divine and overcome
all difficulties. But this is only so long as the higher
Light has not descended into the physical.
-Sri Aurobindo (Ghose, 1996, p. 141).

Humans are in transition: All they need is present,
yet in imperfect order, to degrees involved and asleep.
Hence, the truth of our existence is hidden in the sleep
of deeper structures that can evolve through unfolding
developmental processes— sadhana. When healthy modes
of development are activated, individuals with a reasonably
stable and centralized ego are able to guide their own
personal evolution with some degree of certitude.

On the other hand, for reasons often indeterminable
and other times fairly evident, the centralizing process
of development is fractured. While reasons may be
innumerable, the results present common themes.

Prior to discussing the themes of this fracturing, it is
important to remember that in Sri Aurobindo's view, even
this often tragic state has meaning at the deeper sacred

levels. "The master of our works respects our nature even when he is transforming it; he works always through the nature and not by any arbitrary caprice" (Ghose, 1996, p. 233).

Sri Aurobindo assures us that there is a secret purpose for all states, and that the deeper causative motives may be revealed once fullness has been regained. It is necessary to wake up and to feel the pain, to address the internal and external devastation—the aim is a full and participative force of soul. Therefore, no narrow and mutilated state of superficiality and rigidity full of fear and coldness will suffice. Each difficulty can be faced and mastered, often at different levels of sophistication over time as new skills and attributes unfold (Ghose, 1996).

From this hopeful understanding we can now examine the fracturing effects on the physical, emotional, mental, and spiritual aspects of our nature. In doing so I describe how fracturing the ego can happen from an outer-being perspective, and introduce the role of the inner being while adding thoughts on the role of the innermost being (deepened and refined in later chapters.)

When individuals fracture the outer being's physical, emotional-vital, and mental aspects of self, energy-consciousness-force can be expressed on the physical— as a pathologically induced craving for drugs, food, sleep, material possessions, computer or technological distractions, awards, and a myriad of other desires or affective disorders— such that normal activities of daily living can be subordinated. Illnesses or accidents can occur, along with many emotional disruptions as the interwoven emotional and mental fields gather around specific lead desires. Preoccupation with these desires serves to hold often deeply buried or repressed feelings such as anger, grief, shame, and inner soul-centered pain alongside the conscious and unconscious beliefs that maintain these feelings.

This condition varies in degree with each person,

but serves to fracture and offset egoic development. The fracturing is often initiated at an early age through abuse or trauma, long before the ego is able to develop and stabilize, so that the normal growth and development phases and stages are disrupted. Individuals with a fractured egoic sense of self, just as more or less normal people, long for happiness, equanimity, and an interesting, productive, and meaningful life.

Children learn to cope in different ways. Some are gifted with an amazing resilience, or find at least one person in the world who truly cares for them and who they can trust. This one person may or may not be aware of his or her profoundly positive impact on the child; nevertheless, the caring can sustain resilience so the child manages to cope well enough to develop an egoic view of self on which to build a meaningful life.

Sadly, and all too often, there is no caring person and the abused child learns to cope through a haze of fear, guilt, rage, sadness, and self-blame. Often still functional, the child grows up and can manage—until his or her unstable egoic sense of self is farther fractured through trauma or some catalyzing event. The results are unique to the person.

Depending on the person, this fracturing process impacts the outer-being configurations of consciousness in a variety of ways. In terms of the outer physical, the nervous system and immune and endocrine systems are often compromised, and physical illness or symptoms of dis-ease can manifest, especially when stress is magnified.

The emotional-vital body reacts in two general ways. Rajasic energy can magnify, and hypersensitivity and hyperactivity or agitation and anxiety can occur. In addition, tamas can control the person, and shades of depression can manifest in a wide variety of ways, some more toxic than others. Sometimes there are swings between the tamas and rajasic qualities, resulting in little stability or time for equanimity and recovery to balance.

The outer mental body can hold insight into the issues and causative factors for the egoic breakdown; nevertheless, without impactful strategies to support the coping mechanisms, the physical and emotional-vital rule, and the mental body becomes their slave. This dynamic leaves the door open for other subtle forces to encroach on the healthy potentials that reside internally.

The impact on the inner being shows in the subtle physical and in the emotional-vital and mental parts of the being, which are also fractured, dissociated, and shielded. The human energy field appears torn, distorted, and off-center, often upheld out of the body, fragile and reactive. In many, it is heavily laden on multiple levels with etheric debris. The biofield itself can be compacted and accreted with rage, anger, anxiety, depression, shame, and craving. If this force is imploded internally, it can be held physically in muscle tendons, fascia structures, and organ structures, impacting physiological systems. Though now rooted in the inner being, the disruption emotionally and mentally surfaces as depression, anxiety, fatigue, and feelings and beliefs related to worthlessness and hopelessness, or in lesser states, constant business or preoccupations (Lamb, 2010).

The innermost soul aspect, now often heavily veiled, continues working behind the frontal consciousness in its secret ways. Spiritually, individuals often feel lack of faith and a great inner sadness that is unexplainable. The Mother says that she believes many depressions are not indeed psychological but stem from a sadness of the soul (Alfassa & Ghose, 1999).

From a developmental-hierarchical point of view, the lower planes of consciousness (the inconscient and subconscient) and the lower planes of the physical, emotional, and mental levels of awareness with their unique vibrational frequencies increasingly override the normalizing developmental forces that seek balance and a centralized egoic state. The higher spiritual plane and the innermost soul are present, but to the individual identified with these lower states, they are often too subtle and distant, especially if the disowning progresses.

Not only are there personal inner and outer detractors (including the environmental aspects accompanied by heritage, family, culture, and global impacts), but there are also the hostile occult forces spoken about in the ancient teachings, and surprisingly, written about in modern literature and presented in a variety of ways and styles in postmodern film. In general, Sri Aurobindo speaks of three basic typologies of these forms: the Asura, Rakshasa, and Pishacha, more commonly named in English as Titan, Giant, and Demon.

These occult forces come from the subtle typal (unchanging) and astral worlds, and each form is unchanging and largely focused on a destructive role. The *Asura*, we are told, has great power of thought and holds much vehemence. This presence can have what appear to be moral powers and even appear ascetic and most intellectually persuasive; nevertheless, all outcomes are used for selfish and harmful ends leaving humankind disempowered, disenfranchised, fearful, and robotic. The *Rakshasa* is a cunning ravager ruled by pure greed and the desire for death and ultimate chaos. The *Pishacha*, at an even lower level, seeks and creates torture, aims at all things obscene, and causes much daily disruption (Sri Aurobindo; see Ghose, 1996, 2000c).

In numerous cunning ways, these powers infiltrate the human psyche, take up residence, and lead individuals toward blindness, baseness, lust, greed, anger, rage, and all manner of suffering. What is more, these powers know how to grasp human nature and make it one with the adverse forces; they have done so throughout time.

It is worth remembering these words:

Attacks from adverse forces are inevitable: you have to take them as tests on your way and go on courageously through the ordeal. The struggle may

be hard, but when you have come out of it, you have gained something, you have advanced a step. There is even a necessity for the existence of the adverse forces. They make your determination stronger, your aspiration clearer.
-Sri Aurobindo (Ghose, 1998, p. 142).

As the disowning of self and the fracturing of ego progresses, whether it be a minor fracture in the most normal- appearing person or a major disruption in someone who has never stabilized a reasonable sense of self, openings from the fracturing create a space and opportunity for further destruction—above and beyond the harm we can cause ourselves on our own. Hostile forces, or negative and destructive forms of consciousness that detract from the wellbeing of the planet and humankind, await these fracturing moments. Everyone is vulnerable, and we are assured that we are open to attack whether we are aware or not. The Mother says: "The hostile forces do not need a cause for attacking—they attack whatever and whoever they can. What one has to see is that nothing responds or admits them..." (Alfassa, 1998, p. 141). She goes on to say that "...if one has a complete faith and self-consecration, one can throw off the attack without too much difficulty" (p. 141). These forces working on the side of Ignorance and involution are always ready to bring tamas forward and push rajasic tendencies out of control.

With all great efforts, the Mother assures us, there will be detractions including adverse force interventions. She advises:

To give them too great an importance increases their importance and their power to multiply themselves, gives them, as it were, confidence in themselves and the habit of coming. To face them with equanimity, diminishes their importance and effect in the end, though not at once, gets rid of their persistence and recurrence. It is therefore a principle in Yoga to recognize the determining power of what is within us—for that is the deeper truth—to get that right and establish the inward strength as against the power of outward circumstances. The strength is there— even in the weakest; one has to find it, to unveil it and to keep it in front throughout the journey and the battle. (as quoted by Ghose, 1998, pp. 141-142).

Hope and despair walk side by side. The extent to which hope can override despair depends on how much self-structure or egoic centralization remains activated and can access the secret source of the soul. As we have been assured, there is a deeper soul presence holding hope and waiting for us to receive its profound power, strength, and force of consciousness. The path to soul-presence is nurtured through the development of a centralized ego capable of taking the next evolutionary step toward individuation.

INTEGRAL REFLECTION PRACTICES

We all undergo challenges in life that elicit fracturing; this is natural. However, the most important skill lies in noticing and observing the inner and outer processes that are capable of depleting our resources and detracting from our quality of life, and then using strategic methods to mount an effective response.

1. What experiences are most likely to initiate a fracturing experience?

2. Using your noticing aspects, remember what happens for you in these instances. What do you notice— physically, emotionally, mentally, spiritually, and with your human energy field?

3. What specific sensations are present in your body?

4. What dynamics are present with your conditioned self?

5. Is there a belief underlying your conditioned response? Does the belief still fit? Does it need to be examined further? Can it or should it be changed? If so, what would you like this new belief to look like? Can you name new values that will elicit a new and more evolved belief, and thereby a more appropriate response?

6. Does this reflection elicit a lesson? Word the lesson.

7. Can you sense a deeper, healing response or renewal process underlying the experiences brought to the surface from this example?

5
INDIVIDUATION: ACTIVATING THE FOUR POWERS

This persistent soul-existence is the real Individuality
which stands behind the constant mutation of things
we call our personality....we are not a mere mass
of mind- stuff, life-stuff, body-stuff taking different
forms of mind and life and body from birth to
birth...there is a real and stable power of our being
behind the constant mutation of our mental, vital
and physical personality and this is what me have
to know and preserve in order that the Infinite may
manifest....
-Sri Aurobindo (Ghose, 1996, p. 360).

Individuation—that is, moving Beyond ego—requires
another great work, another dynamic use of the gunas or
qualities of sattwa (enlightened peace), rajas (powerful
dynamism), and tamas (inertia and habit). In individuation,
these gunas are used to express the special power of
soul that organizes itself in the deepest innermost being,
reflecting its light to the inner being and to the outer
being's physical, emotional-vital, and mental nature.

Sri Aurobindo speaks of a four-fold power of
evolution: the power of knowledge and intelligence, the
power of force and strength, the power of harmony and
adaption, and the power of work, service, or labor (Ghose,
1996, 2000c). Each power exists overtly or covertly in all
people, and many claim that the amalgam of these yogic
powers forms a person's character. As the ego strengthens,
centralizes, and learns to overcome the downward pull
from a wide array of adverse circumstances, these powers
refine along with the guna qualities that direct them. When
the ego begins to gain self-awareness, the personality
forms—once a dynamically healthy ego-point of 'I am' is

stabilized, then there is a foundation for individuation.

Once a certain stability has been reached, the ego may be healthy enough to overcome its tamasic inertia, which rests on a refusal to change. The outer emotional-vital ego aspects, having claimed a sense of authority and egoic power on behalf of this 'I', rajasically hold their dominion. Even the outer mental egoic aspect has its challenges with change, once the sattwic quality has developed a standpoint of equanimity with values, beliefs, and doctrine or dogma accepted as right and solidified into a worldview.

Growth beyond the dynamically stabilized ego-point 'I am' requires the force of a more activated soul carrying the spirit of inquiry, a willingness to seek knowledge. A seeking for knowledge and understanding that activates the outer- and inner-mind formations of consciousness. This building of knowledge has innumerable stages, intensities, and maturities. Some individuals remain content with superficial awareness, others seek deeper, and a few will probe to the root of the possible. Without balance, this powerful force of seeking becomes one-dimensional; without practice and integration, knowledge remains theoretical and deadened.

Knowledge and understanding are the first requirements if we wish to achieve, followed by making the knowledge effective. Secondly, strength and will are required, and the ability and courage to carry forth despite obstacles. If knowledge, understanding, and intelligence are not supported by will and strength, the rajasic vital may intervene and destroy the right exercise of power—acute discernment is crucial. Third, there is a need to organize the intelligence and put the wisdom into practice in a wise, co-creative, and harmoniously practical manner. Finally, the fourth power requires that work be done, effort be made, detail be addressed and positive service to humankind be achieved—this is a conscious and surrendered service sustaining dharma, a soul-power which carries meaningful purpose.

As long as the outward personality we call ourselves is centered in the lower powers of consciousness, the riddle of its own existence, its purpose, its necessity is to it an insoluble enigma. -Sri Aurobindo (Ghose, 1996, p. 191).

Individuation requires a person to step away from being directly controlled by the outer physical, emotional-vital, and mental aspects of consciousness and become more awake to the underlying forces that have much greater sway—the inner physical, emotional-vital, and mental. With an active noticing state evolving and the witness consciousness gaining awareness, it becomes possible to seek the deeper, more poignantly urgent forces that subtly uplift manifold suggestions to the outer being. Individuation in this sense means that individuals are becoming just that: centralised in their deeper awareness and capable of greater intelligence in the choices they make. Of course, the outer dynamics and ongoing testing from numerous directions remain; nevertheless, with a healthy enough egoic stance and a willingness to look deeper comes a more directed connection with the innermost being (soul force). This connection itself brings a sustaining stability as faith in something luminous, clear, and wise arises naturally from within, bringing a greater ability to face the fracturing situations that inevitably impact the human condition.

The inner being underlies the outer being and is immersed in a state of subliminal consciousness; therefore, the inner mental, emotional-vital, and subtle physical have a much deeper and broader range of force, power, and consciousness impacting them. Impacts are received from the individual's own history and lifetimes of learning as well as from the environmental and universal consciousness, and from all levels of the hierarchical consciousness. "Our subliminal self...is a meeting-place of the consciousness that emerges from below by evolution and the consciousness that has descended from above for involution" (Ghose, 2000c, pp. 425-427). In order to bring awareness to this domain, it is understandable that the outer egoic self needs to be centralised and somewhat stabilized; then, with a sense of the outer self stabilized, awareness of how much more we are becomes evident as a deeper reflective noticing develops.

> ...our present conscious existence, is only a representative formation, a superficial activity, a changing external result of a vast mass of concealed existence...our existence is something much larger than this apparent frontal being which we suppose ourselves to be and which we offer to the world around us....It is only when we go behind, below, above into the hidden stretches of our being that we can know it; the most thorough and acute surface scrutiny and manipulation cannot give us the true understanding or the completely effective control of our life, its purpose, its activities....
> -Sri Aurobindo (Ghose, 1996, pp. 170-171).

From the inner-being perspective, the inner mind is open to an infinite number of influences from our own subconscient (including access to imprints from our family of heritage and previous lifetimes, from the environment around us, and from those in the environment; In addition, at a collective level (e.g., through the media) many thought forms are impacting individuals globally. Finally, individuals are also impacted by thought forms from the astral and hostile planes as well as from the higher mind, illumined mind, intuitive mind, and innermost soul. The complexities multiply. Each of these mind-related forces of consciousness affects our outer physical, emotional, and thinking mental field.

We have innumerable thoughts each waking moment, and dreams at night—what is real? The main discipline of the mind is noticing, observation, quietening, and controlling, opening to the higher wisdom and receiving that wisdom, all the while using the most acute mental discrimination.

As soon as we can cultivate a soul-awareness, we also cultivate a soul-discrimination—we cultivate what the yogis term the *kshurasya dhara* or the razor's edge.

From an inner emotional-vital perspective the subliminal actively presents waves of life-force and emotional-feeling; hence, when formations from the astral bring imposing and convincing allures forward, being alert is crucial. Sri Aurobindo tells us that the power of the vital formations to flash lights and overwhelm with grandeur and brilliance is dazzling. For example, he says, if a person overwhelms you, pulls you, seduces you, imposes on you, and feeds your ego or your impulse for ambition—you must pull back. A spiritual personality, he says, is nonimposing and strengthening.

The inner vital is connected to and vulnerable to the local and global life force and the emotional streams of innumerable forces and feelings. So, in addition to one's internal pushes and personal feelings poking up from the subconscient and unconscious, this dimension of our being is aware at the consciousness level of the emotional-vital-feeling forces near and far. These waves impact the outer emotional-vital to different degrees in each person, and to different degrees at different times in life. Pandit (1992) tells us that the vital is cunning and convincing:

> Whenever there is an attack or something untoward happens, the ideal way is not to blame others or outer circumstances, but to look into yourself and detect what is false, what is obscure, what is dark in you; and after detecting it, to reject it not only once but persistently because these things have a way of coming back and asserting themselves again and again (p. 14-15).

This process can be carried out from a personal perspective first, then look beyond the self to outer circumstances. For self or others, notice if cunning rationalizations link the lower and higher vital levels, allowing justification of actions that few would condone as right and honorable from an individual or humanitarian perspective. This takes humility, a rather alien attribute to the vital, which is drawn and fed by desire from the lowest level and is capable of sweeping nations into turmoil.

On the other hand, Sri Aurobindo states, the vital is the warrior of the soul—once it is reformed and transformed. Its powerful life force energies and sweeping access to consciousness, tied intimately to emotions and feelings and higher aspiration, can forge the pathway to the innermost being. A keen self-awareness must be cultivated, accompanied by a will for purification through objective self-examination, so that individuals become able to determine the difference between a vital glow or vital glamor, and to identify spiritual radiance. The required skills are based in an ongoing will to change, rejection or refusal of expression based on discernment, and surrender to a call from the soul.

The subtle physical serves to link the outer body physical consciousness to the subtle etheric and astral realms of consciousness, and to the physiological-nervous-system bridge between matter and energy. At the subtle physical, the chakras form an aspect of the bridge and bring subliminal awareness closer to the outer being on the physical, emotional-vital, and mental planes. Sri Aurobindo says that "only a little of the inner being escapes through these centres into the outer life, but that little is the best part of ourselves and responsible for our art, poetry, philosophy, ideas, religious aspirations, effort and knowledge and perfection" (Ghose, 2000b, p. 1165).

The subtle physical holds the body's potential for dis-ease and for health, as illnesses can be held in the human energy field or biofield prior to physical activation. All physiological disruptions pattern into, or arise from, the subtle physical as do all emotional states—they show their legacy within different levels of the human energy field, either as it overextends the physical body or as it lies within the body in the cells and tissues. There may (or may not) be somatic symptoms or a subtle somatic awareness of feeling tones held within the actual tissue structures. As with the inner mental and emotional-vital, the subtle physical interacts with the subconscient, unconscious, and the higher levels of consciousness just as it does with the surface egoic personality and physiological status. This dynamic and interwoven interaction occurring each moment in the moment is detailed in Part Two.

From an Integral yoga viewpoint, individuation becomes a complex process: Step by step, one proceeds by refining the methods Sri Aurobindo and the Mother set forth. For our purposes here, I define the yoga of individuation as

> *the power and the presence, the inner stillness and ability to consciously contact the Inner Guide—the deepest soul awareness—combined with a discerning witness consciousness that allows us to access the highest processes of which our nature is capable; this is a process whereby the inner insight informs the outer sight and is capable of guiding will and action. Here, one is in contact with the innermost consciousness, which is a widened, heightened, and spacious consciousness—a soul- consciousness that reveals the Divine potential in each person and sustains and supports the integration and harmony of all parts of the being.*

This is one view for consideration, but it holds the foundational methods described here and brings understanding to the Integral yoga self-awareness processes. The four powers of knowledge and intelligence, force and strength, harmony and adaption, and work and service are dynamic powers and processes interwoven into the yoga of individuation. The next step functionally is activating the soul. However, at all places and in all instances, the soul is involved—it is a matter of how consciously we as individuals can sustain tapasya, the conscious work of activating soul.

Integral Reflection Practices

1. Reflect on the four powers: Knowledge and intelligence, force and strength, harmony and adaption, and work and service. How do these powers inform your life?

2. From the perspective of the four powers, identify specific circumstances influencing the guna qualities of rajas, tamas, and sattwa that (a) detract from self-awareness and/or (b) elicit self-awareness.

3. Reflect on the yoga of individuation: in what ways do you access your Inner Guide—the deepest soul awareness combined with a discerning witness consciousness? What combination of methods for you is most likely to bring success?

6
Tapasaya: Activating the Soul

Division, ego, the imperfect consciousness and groping and struggle of a separate self-affirmation are the efficient causes of the suffering and ignorance of this world. Once consciousness separated from the one consciousness, they fell inevitably into Ignorance and the last result of Ignorance was Inconscience; from a dark immense Inconscient this material world arises and out of it a soul that by evolution is struggling into consciousness, attracted toward the hidden Light, ascending but still blindly towards the lost Divinity from which it came....
–Sri Aurobindo (Ghose, 1996, p. 191).

All life, spiritual, mental or material, is the play of the soul with the possibilities of its nature; for without this play there can be no self-expression and no relative self- experience. Even then, in our realisation of all as our larger self and in our oneness with God and other beings, this play can and must persist, unless we desire to cease from all self-expression and all but a tranced and absorbed self-experience.
–Sri Aurobindo (Ghose, 1996, p. 419).

Evolutionary tapasya becomes the work of unfolding soul. As the veils encompass the innermost being, the inner being's subliminal consciousness opens to higher and deeper levels of consciousness; outer being awareness develops acceptance of this new illumined knowledge. When differing degrees of conscious awareness occur, behaviors can change to support the evolutionary process, self-reversal occurs as old habits give way to new, more dynamic strategies for living.

Individuals transform aspects of their being as they refine and shift perceptions toward a more aware soul-knowing, and living from within this greater awareness brings a more sophisticated, new integrality. Individuals become more conscious as do the soul forces, or forces of the psychic being as Sri Aurobindo often terms the soul. Outer, inner, and innermost parts of the being interrelate in co-creation.

When it is well established, tapasya pushes forth what Pandit (1994) calls a

> soul-personality, that supports the inner mental, the inner vital and the subtle-physical....And it is this psychic [soul] personality which is turned towards nature that draws the cream of experience and grows. It is intended not only to draw but also to emanate, project the Divine influence on the instrumental nature (p.9).

This process brings the essential self to the forefront and the relative self begins to refine; right effort supported by the soul-personality brings results in daily life. Self-noticing, self- discernment, self-compassion, and self-forgiveness become tools for daily awareness, and there are fewer instances of 'autopilot' causing consternation. The guna tendencies of rajas, tamas, and sattwic ways of being become balanced in a manner that sustains inner development. Pandit (1994) continues:

> One knows that one has a spiritual purpose, a spiritual destiny and one aspires. One puts in effort but after awhile, for whatever reason, possibly due to the pulls of the lower faculties, senses, shadows of the unconsciousness and inconscient, the aspiration flags and one turns back to the little creature comforts, little vital movement of the external way. It is then that the psychic [soul] feels a sadness, because it is unable to influence the material nature; an unaccountable sadness

without any apparent reason, that is the psychic sadness....which [is] altogether on a different plane of experience than the emotional [sadness] (p.10).

The psychic being or soul is a spark of the Godhead veiled in the inner sanctum deep behind our heart space— this soul consciousness remains with us from life to life, developing itself and manifesting more and more as our being ripens. The psychic being activates a longing for the Divine. Its role is to assist humanity's progress toward Divinity, to influence our outer waking consciousness by working with the outward mental being and all its egotistical externalized worldviews. The psychic being attempts to impress itself upon the higher-order emotion of the vital consciousness—to awaken a rather dense physical consciousness, even when the psychic being itself is often steeped in lower-order emotions and desires.

This mostly secret power is hidden behind a veil that can be rent via aspiration or unquestioning surrender to a clearly defined Divine, says Sri Aurobindo (Ghose, 1996). He speaks of the need for constant and sincere aspiration as the key to rendering the veil less effective, thus opening a more consciously aware pathway for the waking consciousness.

Quietude, a sense of peace and calm, a certain silence in the desire heart, purity, and sincerity—all call the psychic being to the forefront. Its presence can increase the truth, power, and intensity of our vision, touch, sense, taste, and hearing. When aspiration is pure, the psychic being guides us to right thought, right feelings, right perception, and right attitude in our outer waking consciousness. It helps us access higher mind and a truer love of the heart. It brings the soul to the foreground in our lives and provides us with opportunities for transcendence. (Sri Aurobindo, see Ghose, 1996).

Once awakened, the soul becomes greatly saddened at attributes such as anger, brutality, arrogance, and other impurities. These negative attributes can initiate an unexplained sadness and push the soul energies into retreat;

moreover, the sadness may turn to depression. Remember the Mother says that living contrary to longings centered in the soul can lead to incorrect labels such as depression or despair, and even a sense of ambiguity or dissociation, clues that aspects of the outer being are off centre for both the healthy centralized ego and the soul (Alfassa, 1998).

Sri Aurobindo says even God cannot change individuals unless they themselves consent to be changed; with this in mind, many traditions have developed methods to activate the inner, sacred source of illumination (Ghose, 1996, 2000c). It is not an easy task, Sri Aurobindo assures us. Each advance is a process and step that may have innumerable fallbacks and regressions; nevertheless, with three admirable qualities in development there is much hope. Three practices, among many others, highly support the unfolding of consciousness that dissolves the veils between self and soul. For our purposes, the three key Integral yoga practices and attributes are aspiration, rejection, and surrender; all have very specific meanings within this context of self-development, and all require the ability to self-gather or centralize the ego, a healthy ego. With self-gathering, the four powers are greatly enhanced.

Finding the key to soul unfolding, according to the teachings, requires sincere and steadfast *aspiration*: a will to call down the Divine source while simultaneously remaining in inner stillness. This 'calling down' and receiving in stillness enables one to remain permeable to the divine Shakti or great manifesting Mother-power. This process requires *rejection*, a complex notion that incorporates witness consciousness, noticing, and a high level of self-discernment—one must be awake in order to make the right choices, at the right time, and in the right manner. The third attribute and practice, *surrender* requires an intricate understanding of wisdom-plus-surrender (certainly not a diffuse, amorphous, naive surrender) and entails a consciousness that can identify the higher luminous consciousness and not be fooled by false renditions. Surrender requires an alignment and plasticity such that the deeper and luminous   consciousness   can teach   and   transform. These attributes are an Integral practice, a tool that supports the call from within and will be discussed in more detail in Part Two.

Elements of aspiration, rejection, and surrender can be consciously applied to life situations. This section offers quotes from practitioners who participated in the research mentioned in the introductory section (Lamb, 2010, pp. 304-305). It takes time to embody depth and soul-centered complexity, and to work through personal surface resistance. During the nine months of the original research study, twelve practitioners participated by offering Integrative Energy Healing treatments in the clinical setting and attended monthly co-creative practitioner- researcher group sessions in addition to several weekend retreats. We were exploring the notion of mystic-scientist- healer or practitioner—examining an expanded integral view of ourselves and our clients. The practitioners' heartfelt insights speak to the tapasya they are undergoing.

For aspiration:

> Edward: I truly want to understand the esoteric teachings of the reality behind the illusion of what we call life, and how the embodiment of such transforms or awakens one into a mystic-scientist-healer. I am having an inkling of what it means to be in on an inner journey. This inner journey must be made, head on, and straight through to the other side. This is my commitment—moment to moment, day by day.

> Xara: The longing in me is to go toward the power of the soul's journey, the authenticity of the soul's decisions regardless of what the ego wants...to know myself profoundly, integrating between higher and lower selves, to learn mystic secrets that surpass all knowledge, to be on the razor's edge, to know the

secrets of healing at the soul's level, to know God. I am longing to find a place of non-judgment and a place where I can trust that everything is unfolding as it should.

For rejection:

Edward: Yes, there are moments when fear is present. As the ground beneath my being continues shifting 'I', my little self, feels threatened. 'I' looks for and comes up with many ways to avoid, postpone, and wish these moments away. At those times when 'I' doesn't feel safe, 'I' remembers there is no choice, and there is protection and guidance.

Joan: There were times during the treatments when I felt like the mother of a vulnerable child needing protection, guidance and love to heal a heart. I wanted to fix things so my clients wouldn't hurt. My training and analytical mind tell me that I can only support them to a limited extent and that I should 'get out of the way' for them to do their own healing work. It was sometimes difficult to do.

Anne: My shadow came up when I wanted to see results immediately, now patience and trust in a Higher Power also matter.

Charlotte: Over the past couple of days I have become increasingly aware of my need to discipline my mind more, and have gained insight into my addictive pattern of indulging my fantasy thoughts to escape my stress. I am being called to be aware of how my intuition and inner guidance can guide my healing of this addictive pattern.

Sophia: It has been interesting as the dark forces have tried in every way to move in since my return home from our retreat. It's like my family member was 'acting out' the internal struggle of weakness that I was experiencing on inner levels of my being.

For surrender:

Sophia: I was challenged to look several of my personal fears in the eye. As a result, I entered the depths. I sense that a huge piece has been surrendered. Identifying these key themes has brought an awareness to discipline myself and wean my ego/personality from the need to recycle. This was an addiction that fed my own emotional jungle.

Xara: I long to fully align with my soul's plan and my life's mission. I believe that my own healing is part of my purpose on earth. I am longing to forgive myself for all the life times that I offended the Divine in any shape or form, in thought or deed and action, and to ask forgiveness.

Joan: There has been a turning point in my faith during these last months, partially due to these [episodes] of unusual assistance and synchronicities during the Integrative healing treatments, and partially due to my longing to connect with my soul.

As these quotes reflect, rejection, aspiration, and surrender are integrally tied to the gunas and the sattwic, rajasic, and tamasic tendencies. The lovely, motivated sattwic longing for a deeper and more aligned existence is often slow to take a steady guidance posture in the psyche; it is far more likely that the rajasic tendencies will push for early success and be intolerant of deviation from the main aim. Impatience is a great stumbling block and a favorite strategy of the rajasic tendencies, as is the tendency to seek everywhere for support versus focusing. Once enough information has been gathered, a person can simply dive and work the tapasya of deepening as would a master woodworker or master musician—diligence and self-mastery have the power to transform an out-of-control rajasic tendency, thereby making an ally with inner development. The tamasic nature has its role as well: It slows us when we are out of control, and it can dampen our zeal quite successfully if it is given too much sway.

The hidden light, we are assured, is present. The eternal Veda (Knowledge) is also present in the deep heart centre; however, the process of human becoming requires work (tapasya), as we are told in many scriptures.

> The eternal Veda is there embedded in the lotus of the heart....Once this store of knowledge in the core of the being starts revealing itself, everything in the outer life, every circumstance becomes an occasion for it. The inner knowledge uses every detail of the outer life to open another page in your being. The same circumstances, the same individuals, the same happenings—if they had taken place, say, five years earlier, or even five days earlier before the inner awakening, would not have carried the same message to you (Pandit, 1999, p. 67).

Part Two presents a perspective on the soul and its powers as this Consciousness, Force, Energy, Light, and Information impact our inner and outer individuality, our karma, and our dharma on this planet.

INTEGRAL REFLECTION PRACTICES

1. Reflect on your experiences of self-noticing and your activation of witness consciousness. In what areas have you gained insight? Journal your reflections.

2. Contemplate issues that have arisen in the process of self-discernment. List a few key issues that are ripe for re-evaluation and reconfiguration in your life.

3. Can you name three areas where self-compassion and self-forgiveness would support your tapasya?

4. Find your own language to express how aspiration, rejection, and surrender can most helpfully impact your life at this time.

PART TWO:
INTEGRAL DIMENSIONS OF CONSCIOUSNESS

7
SUBLIMINAL CONSCIOUSNESS

Our subliminal self is...a meeting-place of the consciousness that emerges from below by evolution and the consciousness that has descended from above for involution. There is in it an inner mind, an inner vital being of ourselves, an inner or subtle-physical being larger than our outer being and nature. This inner existence is the concealed origin of almost all in our surface self that is not a construction of the first inconscient World-Energy or a natural development functioning on our surface consciousness or a reaction of it to impacts from the outside universal nature, --and even in this construction these functionings, these reactions the subliminal takes part and exercises on them a considerable influence. There is here a consciousness which has a power of direct contact with the universal unlike the mostly indirect contacts which our surface being maintains with the universe through the sense-mind and the senses. There are here inner senses, a subliminal sight, touch, hearing; but these subtle senses are rather channels of the inner being's direct consciousness of things than its informants: the subliminal is not dependent on its senses for its knowledge, they only give a form to its direct experience of objects; they do not, so much as in the waking mind, convey forms of objects for the mind's documentation or as the stating-point or basis for an indirect constructive experience.
-Sri Aurobindo (Ghose, 2000c, pp. 425-427).

How are our individual actions—mental, vital, and physical—related to the universal forces? Sri Aurobindo speaks about a multitude of cosmic forces in constant motion, moving in waves and masses capable of affecting all humanity. At the broadest level, these forces influence us through the subliminal planes of consciousness; for example, they influence us via our environmental consciousness, our inner consciousness, or directly at the level of outer mental, vital, or physical consciousness. They have a great power to negatively influence us when they work on our subconscient nature directly, activating seeds of ignorance that will either rise to the surface consciousness or influence us powerfully from the subconscient.

Subliminal forces can be either personal, taking on a personality, or impersonal. Some forces are benevolent, others malevolent, and some are there just to make mischief. These forces contribute to all that goes on behind the veil: Sri Aurobindo (Ghose, 1996) tells us that everything we do is prepared as possibilities behind a veil in a vast, concealed consciousness. We live only on the surface, he reminds us, but our subliminal being observes all.

If we are open to it, the subliminal being will attempt to inform our mental, vital, or physical consciousness via premonitions, attractions, repulsions, intuitions, unexplained warnings, ideas, suggestions, and the like—aiming to increase the negative or the positive. One thing we can consciously know is that, via our unevolved aspects, we can attract what we need to push us through to another level, and we can attract from both the covert and overt worlds of universal energies (Pandit, 1994).

Our growth can be undermined and we can be pressed into challenges of varying degrees that influence our mental, vital, or physical being, or all three; or, on the other hand, the soul can call in a positive experience to wake us up. Where our mental, vital, or physical being is weak, malevolent forces accessing us through the subliminal may attempt to force us into greater ignorance, thereby thickening the veil between the psychic being and our outer consciousness.

We can also seek friendship with some of the forces, for example, those of nature: The Mother (Alfassa, 2005) speaks of creating friends with the conscious entities behind the wind or rain. She also teaches how to increase vital energy by living in harmony with nature and being receptive to nature's energies, thereby building inner power and enhancing our abilities to sustain a higher level of consciousness.

The subliminal consciousness is a vast topic all on its own and worthy of its own text. For our purposes at an introductory level, it is best to focus on how Sri Aurobindo articulates this aspect of the yogic science. What is meant by subliminal consciousness and what is its relationship to our waking consciousness?

The subliminal consciousness resides behind our surface consciousness, behind a 'veil', and is there to support the surface consciousness. Subliminal consciousness has a larger inner mind, emotional-vital, and subtle physical than the more personality-based mind, emotional-vital and physical; it opens to a higher superconscient and to a lower subconscient. This openness means that the subliminal consciousness potentially has access to higher mind, illumined mind, intuitive mind, overmind, and supermind, as well as to the layers of subconscient mind and the inconscience.

The subliminal is supported by the psychic existence or soul existence, and so it can, for example, bring great aspirations forward that support the evolution of humanity. This consciousness is far larger and vaster than the 'apparent frontal being' or outer waking consciousness. Sri Aurobindo (Ghose, 1996, 2000c) states that we can come to know our inner being through accessing the subliminal consciousness. Sometimes called the 'dream self' or 'second body', the subliminal consciousness can open us to the unseen; to our inner visions, past, present, and future; and to other places and planes.

The subliminal consciousness is vast. It holds a huge

force of action, a massive potential within its domain—our busy outward lives can completely obscure its wisdom. Learning to be still enough and clear enough to access it with clarity, surety, and safety is a challenge right at the core of the human becoming process.

From the inner, outer, and innermost being perspective, consciousness is formulated previous to and during conception. Later, as atoms and molecules interact, multiply, and specify, Consciousness, Force, Energy, Power, Light, and Information formulate the embryo and the fetus. Infinite activities take place. Streams of life and light, force and power, and information activate, carrying the child's dharma, karma, and heritage attributes. The mother and father, and grandmother and grandfather for generations all have subtle impact, as do the cultural, global, historical, and immediate environmental influences. All contribute as this little being commits to an earth-life return.

The subliminal consciousness, in effect, interpenetrates all aspects becoming down-gradient aspects of vibratory force, energy, power, light, and information. However, for explanatory purposes here it is considered to be stationed in the inner being, innermost being, and throughout the circumconscient. An amalgamation of infinite numbers of planes or vibrational bandwidths of consciousness, the subliminal consciousness interpenetrates the physical, emotional-vital, and mental on many levels: the unconscious or via the inconscient, the subconscious or subconscient, the conscious and the superconscious (see figures on pages 15 and 21). All occur at varying degrees of impact and with varying degrees of conscious awareness (Dalal, 2001).

As gestation continues, commitments are made at levels beyond our understanding and arrays of choice are encoded; past, present, and future intermingle in a cosmic dance. Much is left to co-creation with Time and throughout time, as infinites dance with infinities—a child is born.

The child, a magnificent being of multifaceted

potential, is born. As Sri Aurobindo writes in *Savitri*:

> Out of the paths of the morning star they came Into the little room of mortal life.
> I saw them cross the twilight of an age,
> The sun eyed children of a marvellous dawn, The great creators with wide brows of calm, The massive barrier breakers of the world And wrestlers with destiny in her lists of will, The labourers in the quarries of the gods, The messengers of the incommunicable,
> The architects of immortality...
> Bodies made beautiful by the Spirit's light... (Ghose, 2005, pp. 343-344).

This child comes with multiple dimensions of potential attributes, and dimensions and planes of Consciousness, Force, Energy, and Light that interact with Information, matter, and time.

From a subliminal view the child is established in present- time but is an outcome of past, present, and future from a nonlocal and yogic perspective. The child is a cosmic energy being of light, force, and love. As the grand design has configured, the outer mental, emotional-vital, and physical form are presented to our outer view— the common view or the materialistic view. Nevertheless, as so many cultural traditions affirm, much more has been activated on levels and planes we are today again attempting to understand and articulate.

This terrestrial evolutionary working of Nature from Matter to Mind and beyond it has a double process: there is an outward visible process of physical evolution with birth as its machinery, -- for each evolved form of body housing its own evolved power of consciousness is maintained and kept in continuity by heredity; there is, at the same time, an invisible process of soul evolution with rebirth into ascending grades of form and consciousness... each life becomes a step in a victory over matter by a greater progression of consciousness in it which shall make eventually Matter itself a means for the full manifestation of Spirit. (Ghose, 2000c, pp. 824-826).

Why did the child come? Why do we come into this existence? According to Sri Aurobindo's teachings on the world- purpose, there is a potential for a spiritual unfolding—this remains a hidden truth underlying all existence (Ghose, 2000c). With this view in mind, the involutionary and evolutionary processes have context.

From his vast yogic experiences, Sri Aurobindo (Ghose, 1996; Dalal, 2001) describes the indescribable by presenting the concentric and horizontal maps of consciousness in order to provide guidance for his metaphysics. They provide much useful guidance, assist in building understanding of the terms of Integral yoga, and present foundational material for this method as practical skills are being developed to address this amazing incarnational gift: human life.

Sri Aurobindo is clear that for humanity to survive, a radical transformation of our human ways is essential. He says

> that there is no other solution that the spiritual cannot but grow and become more imperative under the urgency of critical circumstances. To that call in the being there must always be some answer in the Divine Reality and in Nature. (Ghose, 2000c, p. 1060).

This change requires a spiritualizing of humanity, Sri Aurobindo says:

> Spirituality is a progressive awakening to the inner reality of our being, to a spirit, self, soul which is other than our mind, life and body. It is an inner aspiration to know, to enter into contact and union with the greater Reality beyond, which also pervades the universe and dwells in us, and as a result of that aspiration, that contact and that union, a turning, a

conservation, a birth into a new being. (Saint Hilaire, 1963/2006, p. 51).

Taking Sri Aurobindo's little 'sun-eyed' child (Ghose, 2005, p. 343) as an example, we now know that the subliminal resides behind, below, and around and above the outer mental, emotional-vital, and physical nature. The child's inner mental, emotional-vital, and subtle physical are intimately connected to the subliminal worlds. It can also be seen from Sri Aurobindo's writing that this is a connection with the vast and infinite realms of consciousness, force, energy, and light. Nevertheless, for our purpose (bringing understanding to the process of human becoming in ways that accentuate the support and detractions that can be expected from the subliminal) we use material from my research (Lamb, 2010) to outline parameters and guide understanding.

As children, the adult participants in my research were situated within a subliminal plane of consciousness that included personal human energy field and chakra formations; familial, ancestral, and cultural genetic encoding; and the immediate environment and community as well as the country and global consciousness and force. In addition, solar and galactic energies and archetypal themes set in place throughout historical time, from primitive and primal to pristine and sacred, have impact and interpenetrate with the subliminal plane.

A little girl named Amber from our study frames this discussion. Though blessed with much light as her early childhood pictures show, events intervened that led to an extensive history of trauma. Her genuine desire to heal captured our hearts—as one practitioner stated, "there but for the Grace of God go I."

This little one was birthed into a family that was successful on the outside but rife with alcoholism on the inside— a generational issue of alcoholism and addiction. Her father was an alcoholic and her mother frozen, withdrawn yet aware. Amber was abused by her father from an early age—the father who, when she speaks of him today, brings tears to her eyes as she wonders how she could love someone who would do this to her and who continues to act as if nothing happened.

With nowhere to turn and no one to turn to, the child coped. She learned to dissociate—to leave her body during the traumatic times—thereby splitting the physical, emotional, and mental outer being early. Healthy boundaries were unable to form as was an early egoic sense of person, though a personality did form. As she grew, she learned from the adults that alcohol provides solace and leads to a trance-like state of oblivion. By grade five at ten years old, she was taking high-proof alcohol from her father's still to school in little airplane bottles. Before long she was using marijuana, and as a young teen she frequented bars, pretending to be older. She comments, "I know now that I was a red flag—announcing abuse". She attracted much more abuse.

If only—yes, if only—someone she loved and respected had been able to reach the younger child before the damaging split that fractured much of the centralizing required for ego development. Her child-strategies leaned heavily on the subliminal inner being: She dissociated, left her body, and found an alternative calm space where she could feel safe. She developed clairvoyant or extended seeing powers that caused her, as a young child, to see into the subliminal realms, noting images that she did not have the tools to understand. This experience increased her need for alcohol, which served to block and deaden an energy field that had porous boundaries, allowing far more of the subliminal to enter than she had the ability to cope with. This 'sun-eyed' child Sri Aurobindo speaks about was being sacrificed to the lower, coarse, and crude demanding world of adult desire.

Imprisonment was ripe, a natural consequence. Alcohol, and other hostile forms and forces, family history and family trauma complemented with narrow views of desire and narrower views of how to find solace created a tragedy in the making. Redemption comes with widening the view, understanding the forms imprisonment can take, and developing strategies— warrior-hero strategies that can uplift individuals and bring a purified solace. Such solace lasts through time and plants seeds that encode new behaviors 'initiated' in the inner being and manifested in the outer being.

Amber's strategies were similar to those of the other adults in the study who themselves had experienced childhood abuse. The outer-being physical, emotional-vital, and mental were under severe threat, and the small children were dependent on adult caretakers. Being so small, they had not yet gathered enough force, energy, and information to form the egoic structure that may have led them to seek assistance elsewhere. Their strategies tapping into the subliminal included dissociation (disappearing from self and placing consciousness and energy in the subtle body on the subliminal plane) and clairvoyance.

An opening of extended vision, especially to the realms of the subtle physical and inner emotional-vital, clairvoyance allows children to 'read' their environment. They mostly 'read' through noting the inner realms' colors around their caregivers, instinctively knowing which colors meant danger. One participant, using precognitive skills, knew ahead of time when his father would arrive home and which evening would mean beatings or when his sisters would be abused. On those days, he stayed out of sight as much as possible; nevertheless two or three "beats a week" was the tragic normal in that house. Another boy, when placed in the small cupboard where his mother kept her liquor, not only left his body but learned how to enter the astral field and travel around the house. He notes that he frequently saw other images floating in the house, which would scare him back into his body.

Dissociated states accompanied by clairvoyant vision

can be terrifying or solace-sustaining, depending on which realm the child enters. Some access frightening forms, and others speak of feeling supported. One physician shared that she only survived because she left her body and was embraced by the light during the dark rituals she was subjected to as a child. She not only felt surrounded by light, she felt her own brilliant soul light activate and remain steadfast inside the centre of her being—an example of the innermost being stepping forth, a soul presence.

The subliminal plane provided children with access to survival strategies, whether positive or negative. Because of fracturing and porous boundaries between the inner and outer being, the subliminal world was able to filter through—at first, during times of trauma, and later during times of stress or high anxiety. As the ego continued to fracture and self-blame and shame escalated, the worlds or planes started to interpenetrate daily activities. Because trauma is associated with the lower realms and coarser energy, the breakthroughs brought frightening visions from the subtle physical and negative story- lines filled with self-blame from the inner and outer emotional-vital and mental realms.

Our clients, wounded early, suffered extremes in their subliminal breakthroughs to the outer being. Porous boundaries led to interpenetration of the lower subliminal and subconscient, causing the desire to self-negate and seek self-solace through alcohol or drugs. Many addictions may stem from some conscious or unconscious running away—a refusal to address dimensions that interact with all of humanity. Given our present-day lack of awareness or lack of courage to address these multiple realms, it is not surprising that those with unusual sensitivities and the special gifts of extended senses feel unsupported, misunderstood, and perhaps stigmatized into silence. Their experiences may or may not include repression, fear, and the need to take substances; or conversely, they may rajasically fill each moment of life such that distraction overrules the upwelling subliminal awareness.

Chapters particularly in Part Three discuss the beauty and illumined support sustained within the subliminal as it opens to the higher illumined, intuitive, and overmind, and as it deepens and embraces the innermost soul-processes that open the way to the sun-lit path. First, however, a powerful contextual understanding of the emotional-vital is needed, supported by graphic experiential sharing in order to link theory to practice and concepts to life. Being-in-the-world, let us embody the wisdom that supports healing potential with eyes wide open.

8
Emotional-vital Body Consciousness

From the life-part of us, the desire-part is being always touched and influenced; there too are beneficent and malefic powers of good desire and evil desire which concern themselves with us even when we are ignorant of and unconcerned with them. Nor are these powers merely tendencies, inconscient forces, nor, except on the verges of matter, subconscient, but conscious powers, beings, living influences. As we awaken to the higher planes of our existence, we become aware of them as friends, or enemies, powers which seek to possess or which we can master, overcome, pass beyond and leave behind.
-Sri Aurobindo (Ghose, 1996, p. 434).

In many ways the power-house for transformation or destruction, the emotional-vital is equally capable of manifesting truth or falsehood. If it is made the master of one's being, it can rule desire-nature with an iron fist; materialism will be its consort and a rampant gathering or longing for glamor, possessions, objects, experiences, or happenings will lead the consciousness. When it is transformed into a servitor of the soul and of higher mind, the emotional-vital becomes the warrior of truth, compassion, wisdom, and right living—an advocate for unity and higher dharma, or right action.

Throughout human history, people have formed ideas as to how dharma to right action can overcome the powers of falsehood. Cultures select their perspectives, with many cultures turning what was not understood about this tension into superstitions. Sri Aurobindo shares his view on this pull towards falsehood and the realm of supra-material:

It is this possible relation of the human being with the powers of the life-world which occupied to so large an extent European occultism, especially in the middle ages, as well as certain forms of Eastern magic and spiritualism. The "superstitions" of the past, -- much superstition there was, that is to say, much ignorant and distorted belief, false explanations and obscure and clumsy dealing with the laws of beyond, --had yet behind them truths which a future Science, delivered from its sole preoccupation with the material world, may rediscover. For the supra-material is as much a reality as the existence of mental beings in the material universe. (Ghose, 1996, pp. 434-435).

We ask, what does this complex interference look like from an outer emotional-vital-being perspective? Steeped in desire, sensations, emotions, and passions with their underlying sets of feelings, the outer emotional-vital energy body holds much power.

Within this schema, the emotional-vital with its multiple dimensions has been divided into three main forms by Sri Aurobindo (Ghose, 1996). The lower vital-physical instinctive nervous-system response rules much of the outer being and physical body. For example, in many cases fight, flight, or freeze responses activate before the mental thought process can intervene. The middle emotional-vital focuses on needs, wants, and a range of feelings such as fear, greed, envy, jealousy, anger, rage, and so on. The higher vital holds ideals, imaginations, and values that—once purified—ensure the vital becomes an ally toward realization. Without purification, these powerful ideas can be used to support the ego in self-serving ways. In addition, underlying the outer realm, the inner being emotional-vital is steeped in feeling-based subconscient material held within the wider-ranging subliminal consciousness.

Consider how these aspects of the emotional-vital interrelate and impact individuals who have experienced risk, trauma, or fear and uncertainty—after a time they are primed to enter a protective mode of fight, flight, or freeze at the merest hint of uncertainty. The perceived degree of uncertainty, accompanied by the perceived degree of risk, provides an instant response from long held grooves of consciousness. These grooves are held in place by the chakra system and the nervous system, and originally coded there by the emotional-vital being at all three levels (more will be said on this when we discuss the physical body consciousness.)

Given the outer emotional-vital has a hypersensitive coding for fight, flight, and freeze, what might happen if someone has been unable to centralize the ego and develop a fairly stable and unified personality? Reaction is rapid, there is no understanding, no time to discern new responses.

Sri Aurobindo speaks of the many personalities within each of us that contribute to human existence: "Even in the human being there are many personalities and not only one, as used formerly to be imagined; for all consciousness can be at once one and multiple" (Ghose, 2000, p. 382). For our purposes in describing how the emotional-vital can influence a person's life, these "many personalities" are termed *subpersonalities*— personalities that have constellations of energy crystallized to differing degrees yet separate from the main personality. Given the right incentive from the emotional-vital, the subpersonalities drive different aspects of daily existence. Specifically, here we examine selected subpersonalities that have formed in individuals who have been unable to centralize an egoic structure, and therefore have not formed a dynamic personality to support growth and development in a reasonably normal manner.

The *healthy ego*, as we are defining it, is the ability to centralize a sense of self such that the many aspects of self can adhere together under a surface personality that depicts the basic nature of the person. This centralization requires, at minimum, a reasonable interweaving of the outer physical, emotional-vital, and mental aspects of the being. When individuals are traumatized, the developing ego is fractured to differing degrees depending on the severity of the trauma and the innate characteristics of the individual. Early traumatic wounding can and often does stifle the natural developmental tendencies, as depicted by the large split in the image "Fractured Ego".

Fractured Ego

Almost all the clients in my research spoke of childhood trauma, which appears to have hindered egoic development and allowed splits in the psyche—a fracturing of the ego admitting confusion and chaos, and depleting a sense of centralizing and stability in the formation of the 'I'. A number of clients asked with poignant agony, 'Who am I?', because the usual patterned energy configurations or subpersonalities began deconstructing when clients immersed themselves in the addiction treatment centre therapies and in the integrative healing research. However, it takes time, personal choice, and support for the new, centralizing understanding of who they can be to stabilize.

A new analysis of the research from the lens of subpersonality shows that as clients shared their stories, subpersonalities were evident: crystallizations of energy in a constellated form, powered by the emotional-vital (Lamb, 2010). The formation of subpersonalities is complex and there is much more to be understood from Sri Aurobindo's notion of multiple personalities, but within this study, clients formed subpersonalities that consisted of a dual nature. They were subject to either aspect of the duality; however, most clients utilized one aspect of the subpersonality while the other was in shadow. In order to cope with early childhood trauma, certain survival techniques were required and these techniques overrode the normal formation of the ego and centralizing of a personality structure to support growth and development.

The dual-sided subpersonalities noted in this study are victim-child versus abuser/bully-child; responsible-child versus rebel-child; carefree child versus fearful child; unlovable-child versus sorrowful/depressed child;

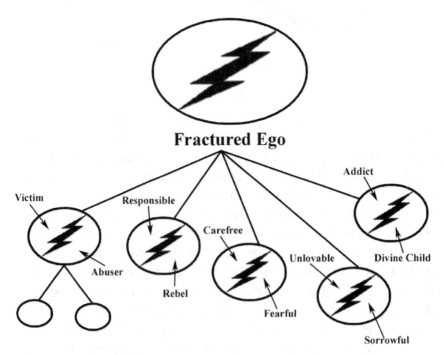

Fractured Ego and Subpersonalities

and addict versus divine-child. These subpersonality constellations of energy with power and focus can work for or against the client, and for or against others: clients can switch to the shadow side of the duality and use it for or against themselves or another. Both sides can be considered shadow; however, there seems to be internal connections between certain emotion-states. The overriding theme with each client was that degrees of childhood abandonment of nurturing and caring by the parents were accompanied by trauma, whether physical, emotional/mental, or sexual. The initiating factor for addiction in the study appears to stem from childhood wounding (Lamb, 2010).

The original research analysis examined the 'coming apart' and the 'coming together' processes as stations of awakening (Lamb, 2010). This view delves into the concentric and hierarchical flows of consciousness as individuals deconstruct and reconstruct the human condition in ways that build bridges toward human becoming. In gratitude to the clients and practitioners who participated in the study and to the amazing co-creative work they did together, this text shares findings that honor childhood and the role of early abuse as it impacts addiction.

There are numerous angles from which to discuss subpersonalities, and there are innumerable subpersonalities. The following micro-stories from the research display how subpersonalites identified in this research influence clients. Researcher comments and client and practitioner abridged quotes are included (Lamb, 2010).

Once the ego fractures, aspects of the child's wounded nature split—at times, these splits host a dual nature. Here we consider each split and its duality as shown in the image below. All quotes are from Lamb (2010, pp. 110-205), with page number indicated; some material is slightly abridged.

Victim-child versus abuser-child

Owen, at 19 our youngest client, struggles with a troubled childhood that included bulimia as well as addiction and issues with being gay. According to a drug and alcohol counselor who is also a sexual assault counselor, he may also have been molested by a man when he was around eight or nine years old. He did not mention this. Owen tells us that it is rare for someone so young to seek treatment. His decision came as he drew close to suicide. He speaks of his addictions:

> Yah, that was my first addiction, food and uh then bulimia. It started when I was 15, cause I used food to uh, to stay fat I didn't want to have relations with girls, but in the end I was an emotional eater. Then I decided to come out and lost 30 pounds but that was not fast enough so the only way to do that was to purge...

When asked if he used drugs to get rid of the feelings of shame and of being different he had spoken about earlier, he replied:

> Ahum, oh yah. I ate them and then I drugged them away, very simple...um simple equation for me. I probably drank less than most of my friends but marijuana hit a chord with me...it made me not want...I didn't want to think about my body. I also used Ritalin in grade twelve. I was snorting it quite a bit, got it from a student [who had a prescription]. Um, I'm going to...going to...um definitely need alcohol. I don't know if we're done, um, I'm worried about that. I work its great money...I make eleven thousand dollars within three months. I have nothing at all at the end of it because I go out and buy like a quarter or an eight a day, forty to fifty bucks of uh pot, weed, all of them, marijuana...and then if I go out and buy alcohol on top of that. They have an interesting um relationship...with weed it—almost

every moment of the day I want to be high. This all started around 17.

One postulates that here is a wounded-child subpersonality holding shame from an early age as he had shared how different he felt from the young age of about eight (p. 247). Owen said:

> So at some point the consequences became too much for me to bear...I really did want to die. I didn't want to take my life so much and I would go through certain um like I would put the belt around my neck, but never you know, try to choke the life out of myself. Just...I was inching closer and closer...and I felt my life was in danger.

Owen had been placing his belt around his neck for some time usually when he was feeling paranoid and uncertain. One day he realized that he was making the belt tighter and tighter. This awareness led to his call for an ambulance and request to be admitted to the psychiatric unit of a hospital for treatment. After some weeks in the hospital his parents suggested addiction treatment. He went straight from the hospital to the treatment centre where we met him.

The outer emotional-vital, as seen in this model, was being empowered by some fractured aspect or subpersonality—a victimizing shame and self-hate intertwined. Over time as the belt got tighter, Own enjoyed the feeling of almost losing consciousness. It was a spark of insight and a deeper, more healthy awareness—even perhaps honor and love for the self— that led to Owen reaching out and obtaining assistance. In treatment he addressed many of the issues that led to his addiction. Nevertheless, before he completed the research he attended a family funeral, and after that in an interview mentioned that he had had one alcoholic drink after the funeral. He said that he still wanted to drink as it related to having fun, but acknowledged that alcohol was his gateway drug to marijuana. He did not return for his final session with the practitioner, and he did say that he did not think he was finished with the addictive lifestyle he was choosing. Insight is present, just not powerful enough to drive this recent lesson home. Nevertheless, given his basic understanding, perhaps time will bring healthier choices.

Owen provides an example of the victim versus abuser duality. Initially victimized by parents who were homophobic, he took on their view of homosexuality and then in turn victimized himself. Initially overeating to fill his every need, he then became bulimic in reaction. In addition, he used marijuana and alcohol to enable a state that abused others.

Owen speaks about the drugged state that gives the abuser subpersonality leeway (p. 126):

Owen: It's a different kind of fun. It's a fun... um... uninhibited fun. It uh...I don't even...I mean, looking at it, "what kind of fun is it?" It's uh, it's hmmm...it's fun where I don't have to think about what I'm going to say or I don't have to have feelings about what I've said. You know um...I don't have to care if someone says something rude to me. I don't have any emotions when I'm drunk and I wouldn't say I am cold. I'm very, very kind but I have...it's very black and white. I'm very either kind or I'm very cold and vicious. And I love that. I am not a fighter or anything, my mouth is just...I spit daggers [laughter] and I don't know, I guess that's part of what alcohol does. I'm definitely the facilitator, I definitely enjoy it.

Ruth: You enjoy it, but is it you or just a force going through you?

Owen: Ummm, I think it is both...it's mixed...

Finally, in order to seek a way out of this victim-abuser state while high on marijuana and alcohol, he sadly turned to his belt and a slow process of self-oblivion. Fortunately he had enough of an egoic structure and maturity combined to call for assistance.

Samuel's experience shows another aspect of the victim-child versus abuser-child subpersonality. In this particular schema Samuel brings a third aspect, warrior-child, into his life as he states he recalls being a warrior in past lifetimes and sees a vision of himself dressed as a warrior in medieval times.

As a very little boy, Samuel (now in his early 40s) remembers having plywood placed over his crib by his parents so they could go out and work on the farm. Samuel speaks: "Like, my whole childhood was kind of taken from me, pretty much." Samuel is sipping alcohol from his father's still at five years old, has alcohol poisoning as a young teen, drinks and smokes marijuana regularly, and then moves on to many street drugs. Later he turns to crack, which becomes impossible to stop (p. 108).

Ruth: Your childhood was pretty traumatic? (p.139)

Samuel: Oh yeah. And I got a lot of beats, though. Like, for stupid things like getting my snow boots wet inside, you know. Getting them off and hitting me with them over the head, you know? I remember getting this peanut butter jar getting broken over my head, like at the age of probably two or three because I had done something. I got beats probably three or four times a week.

Samuel went on to share how he only can think of his hate for his father. Then he says that he has in some ways outdone his father in deeds, just different deeds; this is said with distain for himself. In his surpassing his father's deeds he has been in jail and considers himself very lucky to be alive. Now he wants to develop his skills and move on to a different life style.

Samuel's subconscient saw everything, missed nothing, and interpreted all actions in its own manner, locking his consciousness into imprisoned bundles of perceptions held within the inner and outer being. The victim-child coped on the surface, and when Samuel was under the influence of drugs, the shadow abuser-child was easily activated: the abuser-father was mirrored, and the son a victim of his childhood. Nevertheless, Samuel now knew, at least cognitively, that he had to overcome his history.

Responsible-child versus rebel-child

Ted, another client, is aware of one of his split-off subpersonalities, which he named the 'Reckless one'. The other side of this constellation has been named the responsible-child (Lamb, 2010, p. 116).

A man in his 60s, Ted seemed to be coping well with some drug usage until a family catastrophe occurred followed by a divorce. When he speaks of his childhood, which he does not seem to like doing, he mentions the fact that he had to be very responsible. When asked if there was alcohol or drugs in the family, he says his mother managed his father's alcohol very well. Currently, he is close to his mother; his father died some time ago. Ted speaks of his succumbing to the slippery slope of addiction: to becoming "a scrambled mess." Ted shares:

> Oh yeah. But 'he' convinced me that that was the way to go when you want to shut out the pain. If the smart one had been in control, he wouldn`t have done that. He would have got rid of his baggage and then got rid of the pain. Not try to hide from it...I drank and then I didn't drink for ten years. And then I drank. And then one day I thought, I drink too much, No, you are just going to have one beer. It is okay to go to the bar, but one beer. And that was fine. So I was able to control that. But the drugs...

> when I lost my daughter and I lost money and I lost
> a lot of other things, I was broken down. That was a
> hard feeling to describe losing her. [Ted discovered
> his teenage daughter. She had hung herself.] It was
> like a limb of my chakra cut off leaving my energy
> to drain out. I couldn't hold it in. I was awake all of
> the time.

This led to progressive use of cocaine, crack, and finally
some crystal meth. Ted realized it was death or recovery
for himself. He chose recovery.

In this example, Ted knew when his 'Reckless
one' personality stepped forward from having thoroughly
listened to it for some time. He came near to losing his
business and his house before he gathered all his strength
and requested assistance and treatment. Even now, well
on his way to recovery two years later, though clean, he
speaks of the 'Reckless one' that tempts him from time to
time. He says he needs to keep that part of him, but 'he'—
his more centralized self—must always stay in charge.

When asked if he was ready to release this reckless
aspect of himself, after reflecting, he was clear that he
did not wish to do so; it was part of him, just not a part
that could be allowed to rule his behavior. This holding on
could be an example of the rajasic ego stubbornly refusing
to release the self-destructive constellation. Somehow,
Ted may feel that it empowers him—certainly it holds the
power to destroy. It is also a sign that he may not have
healed and integrated the childhood wound that led to the
rebel-responsible subpersonality split.

In this example the responsible-child subpersonality
held sway during his childhood with some shadow aspects of
the rebel-child intruding. However, Ted says he maintained
a responsible-son perspective throughout childhood and
appears to have considerable maturity, enough to hold
a centralized ego in place. It was not until stress and
tragedy combined on many fronts that resistance fell and
the shadow aspect of the responsible-child was released

as the rebel-child was highly empowered. These repressed emotional-vital forces so long held in control were about to take Ted to the grave through using cocaine, alcohol, and crystal meth.

Ted names the aspect of himself that took him into addiction (Lamb, 2010, p. 151).

> Ted: I took crystal meth to get off crack. And I knew the dangers of it. I knew that I could use the one for the other to get rid of the other one because I had to wait so long to get in here. [5 months.] I knew when I got here, I knew I needed more. I have been out of control for a long time, three years. Now I have my control back.

> Ruth: What does out of control mean?

> Ted: I was fully in control of what I was doing all of the time, right. But [it was] not the person that`s in control right now.

> Ruth: Who was in control?

> Ted: The other me. I guess it would be breaking down my personalities. The reckless personality was in control. Yeah. But 'he' convinced me that drugs were the way to go when you want to shut out the pain. If the smart one had been in control, he wouldn`t have done that. He would have got rid of his baggage and then got rid of the pain. Not try to hide from it.

> Ruth: So the Reckless one gave you the tools for hiding.

> Ted: Yeah. I understand that one part of our personality starts in the womb, right. That's even

> from the voices you hear and the other things. And then there's the other, the rational. And then there's the reckless one. But it is not good when the reckless one takes control. So I have usually been in control and occasionally that guy pops up...When Andrew, my friend came here, he was a disaster. He was just uncontrolled energy, out of focus. I was just a scrambled mess. I hate to think about how I am now to what I was ten weeks ago. Horrible.

The Reckless one takes over and rules, leaving a "scrambled mess," as Ted describes himself. Ted (he contacted me after the research period ended) is still hearing the voice of the Reckless one. He says this personality of the addict, as he calls it, is sly and sneaky and tries to bribe him with promises. Even now, two years later, he also wants to keep "that guy there [within him]".

The responsible-child makes attempts to manage life, but without a strong, adult, centralized ego support, the rebel escapes. What is more, the rebel-child is present in the covert environment of the home and may influence family dynamics. In his insistence that this part of him is required, the mature Ted seems to know that the rebel-child holds a gift; however, as long as the rebel-child is held in place by the wound, its gift is hidden and its dangerous side resides in the subconscient lower emotional-vital, never far from the surface.

Carefree-child versus fearful child

Julia is on the alert, with some inner antennae always poised to warn her about her inability to meet expectations—for her, drugs brought solace and carefree moments (Lamb, 2010, pp. 130-131).

> Julia: It's hard for me to relax. It's so hard for me. Why is it so hard? Because I have to be alert all of the time and paying attention to everything that needs to be done or taken care of and if I let down

my guard, something's going to go wrong in my life.

Ruth: Did that happen when you were a little girl?

Julia: I guess. I don't know. Like, I'm scared to let down my guard. Like, if I laugh and have fun it's to get myself in trouble. It's like, if I'm not watching everything all at once, then something's going to go crazy. Something's going to fall apart. I have this fear that I can't just be carefree and not think about stuff. It is fear of everything, ungrounded and unfounded fears.

Ruth: And you take things to kill all of those fears. What creates them?

Julia: Yeah. An inability to face life on life's terms. Not taking responsibility. Being stunted in the age you were when you first started using. Those are some of the reasons. You've not had a lot of experience with dealing with life in reality because if you've been using for some years of your life you've been avoiding really, seriously coping with life properly and anaesthetizing yourself. And they create a lot of dysfunctional relationships and chaos. And throw into that mess a religious background where it was like, "God's going to get you" or whatever. So there's those fears. Fear of going broke because you've wasted all your money on drugs or alcohol. Fear that you're partner's going to leave you because you're drinking. Just fear, fear, fear, fear everywhere. Not knowing how to deal with life. No life skills because since the person was 13 years old, they've been using drugs to take care of every problem.

Ruth: Was it for you?

Julia: Yeah. 13. Then at 14 I smoked pot. In grade 9, I was smoking pot all the time. I smoked pot constantly. And then I quit pot and I just started drinking when I was 15 and then I started working when I was 17. I worked full-time ever since then. Just went out and drank on the weekends, and not every weekend. Like, I could go without drinking but then the pressure would build up. You know the stress of trying to function as a normal person. I wasn't like a normal person. So I would just go out and get drunk because I needed to de-stress and that was my way of doing it because I'm not really like regular people—just haven't been really responsible.

At times, Julia expresses herself from the third-person point of view—perhaps making it safe by generalizing. Drugs became useful 'anaesthetizing' agents. She speaks of how well they address her anxiety, and how they have made her life manageable and provided her with some carefree times of ease. Of course, that is, until life became unmanageable with them.

Luke states that he used drugs to escape fear and imploding anger (Lamb, 2010, p. 131). When he uses, he says, he lives in a 'fog' and is calm; in addition, drugs reduce the fear that he says was initiated when he was a child.

Ruth: Fear was part of what was drugged, up in the fog? Some of the drug taking reduced anger?

Luke: Yeah. Because people said that, "You're kind of opposite." Because I'd do the drugs and I'd just be calm. When I wasn't using, that's when I was really irritable. And I do get scared. Like this scared feeling all the time. Not all the time.

Luke swung between from calm and fogged to being irritable, fearful, and angry. He used more and more, and finally a life- threatening too much.

Paul expresses the carefree-fearful dichotomy in another way. He states that as a child he had constant feelings of unease, was "pain-stricken", and had a feeling of being apart— versus the carefree feeling he had when he took drugs. His mother died in a car accident when he was a young baby, and his father was an alcoholic that frightened his son with his outbursts of anger (Lamb, 2010, p. 132).

Paul told me how the early alcohol use eased his discomfort, brought solace, and made him feel better. It helped him cope with the feelings that he was apart from society and, for a time, kept him successfully "out of the now". People would ask Paul about his family, and as a small child he was unprepared; he had been given no tools to help him respond in a way that felt clear for him.

> Paul: I was never comfortable as a kid and it caused...I was just emotionally pain-stricken from these things, so I would quickly change, fantasize or just avoid that at all cost if I could. But it was just that constant emotional struggle and things weren't really explained...were never really explained to me as a child. And my grades suffered for it and I was very shy as a child. I started using drugs at an early age and alcohol. I remember looking forward to opening dad's beers as early as five, six or seven and having the first little sip out of it before I took it out of the kitchen on Saturday morning. And by grade four, I was smoking cigarettes and drinking sherry with my nanny. That was a little bonding thing. We had Tuesday night's Red Skelton and Paul Jackson cigarettes and sherry.
>
> Ruth: Grade four, cigarettes and sherry with the nanny?
>
> Paul: Tuesday night. That was our big night. I looked forward to that as a child. And by grade six I started purchasing my first hashish and it just sky-rocketed.

I never used to go home on weekends. I was in a private school in grade six and going to friends' houses, it was very easy to acquire alcohol. And most of the boys that I went to school with shared the same...alcohol, hash and marijuana.

Ruth: So what would you reach that required you to keep wanting to take it? What state did it give you that was so useful?

Paul: It took me out of now. It got me out of the way I was feeling right there and then. And if it worked, I took it. It took out me out of reality and...like I say, I was very uncomfortable as a child and it made me feel better and made me forget for a while...I loved drugs as soon as I experimented with them.

The drugs act as rescue agents or solace-agents, and appear—at least initially—to be the answer. They cover up pain, anguish, feelings of despair, and any sense of undeserving and self-blame. For Paul, drugs "anaesthetize," "de-stress," take clients "out of the now," and make them overall "feel better" so they can have that moment of peace and calm or a high, thereby eliciting an ultimately false, transient, yet sought-after forgetful, fogged state.

The natural desire for freedom, fun, and release is present in us all—it is normal. Simply the desire to be with what is, without overlays imbedded in anxiety, is natural. However, for Julia, Paul, and Luke there were no carefree moments free of the overlay of fear without the drugs. Fear was engrained into the consciousness, stacked on multiple levels of the outer and inner being. They took the by-pass route offered by drugs until drugs, too, failed.

Unlovable-child versus sorrowful-child
Amber felt unlovable unbearably early. We spoke about her sense of self (Lamb, 2010, pp. 134-135).

Amber: I am distorted on the body image and the beauty and sex and love and all that stuff. And I know, by knowledge only, that if someone truly loves you it doesn't matter what you look like and it doesn't matter about your body parts or your physical appearance because love is supposed to be from within. But the rest of it...I don't know. It's not there yet. It's like I've been in a war.

Ruth: Loving yourself, opening your heart to yourself.

Amber: That's the hardest part of everything. That's the part I'm still trying to get. If I can be kind and loving to myself and then I've got to quit taking on people's negative energies and owning other people's stuff and concentrate on me and get my own boundaries and my own strength. Not bad walls, but good walls. Even when my boyfriend left the other day, and he paid me less money than he owed me because he didn't want to break the bills because he wanted them for dope. And he left instantly. And it was like a huge kick in the gut because I just thought he would have liked me more or cared for me more. And then I had the little war with myself. "I'm not good enough. I'm too ugly." I think about the addiction part where it overtakes everything.

Amber notices and takes on the energy of those around her and seems to easily place herself in harm's way, both in terms of self-harm and external risk-taking behaviors. She intellectually knows it is good to offer self-love, but cannot yet internalize the sense or embrace the needed behaviors. Amber shares how self-destruction to her physical body in some way reaffirms her unlovability.

Ruth: Are you still having nightmares?

Amber: Yeah. I wake up lots in the night. I have flashes of different abuse that was done upon me.

And I developed, about 11 years ago, a picking disorder where I actually pick my skin and I would wake up picking at myself. I wake up doing that. Or if I'm feeling really cruddy I just go to the mirror and then I start and I can't stop. It's almost like slashing. I've got whatever they've got wrong. But I just do it in a different form. I can't remember really what happened eleven years ago but I just went into that trance and I picked my face so bad for the first time that I couldn't actually go out of my house for like a week. I didn't go to work. I didn't leave. I had to get aloe vera plants and hydrogen peroxide and heal. And now I have a whole routine of picking and healing, which is pretty pathetic. Do you understand that?

Ruth: I hear you.

Amber: I would wake up fighting for my life, type of thing. I sleep with a baseball bat. And I've slept with a baseball bat for many years. If it's not in my bed, it's close to my bed. Close to around me. And I asked if I was allowed to bring my baseball bat and they said no. And I had a lot more anxiety. So I was doing all these day programs so I could go home to my house at night and feel safe. And then because the insurance company heard the word "cocaine" and they twisted it so...In one way I'm kind of grateful, though, now, because I did learn a lot here in treatment. And I was safe here, so it was actually a good experience in that way.

Ruth: Your body had an experience of being safe and cared for without the bat.

Amber: Yeah. Like they said, you had your own room with a lock on it. And the first couple of days I was really wary and then it's almost like you went to the opposite where I didn't really want to leave. But I am damaged goods here. Like, just the obliteration and the fogginess and the craziness of my head. I wrote down all the sexual abuse and the rapes and the torture and the stuff that has happened to me. And I'd never said it all.

Feeling unlovable, Amber speaks of her previous partner, of "things he's physically done to me and mentally done to me. Those were crimes all by themselves and he should have gone to jail, or could have gone to jail if I would have reported them." Amber allows a reinforcing of her unlovability.

Here we see how pervasive the sense of unlovability is and how sorrow-filled Amber is about how others treat her, and how she treats herself. As we saw in the previous chapter, Amber was abused by her father from a young age and stated that her mother was aware of the abuse. Her sisters are presently addicted as are her whole extended family; she was the only one clean at the spring family gathering she attended.

John has shared how he feels unlovable. He told me he was asked to leave his foster home at age sixteen (Lamb, 2010, p. 139).

> John: Yeah. I went to live with a legal guardian because I wasn't getting along with my (adoptive) parents.
>
> Ruth: So were you...somehow you left that house feeling that you weren't lovable, you said earlier. You had a difficult childhood then?
>
> John: I would say. I had a difficult time relating with my parents and I would go through what my mother calls "slumps" where my life would fall apart even when I was 10 or 11, as much as a 10- or 11-year-old

can fall apart. Then I would have to work my way back up again.

Ruth: How can a life fall apart? How did you fall apart?

John: Emotionally, I guess. I would just... It would snowball. I would get in trouble around the house or...I wasn't a bad kid. I never started using until I was like 17. There were a lot of little rules and stuff at the house and once I started feeling down or something I would just not be mindful of a lot of things. Or have a bad attitude or...

Today, John still feels that he "wasn't a bad kid," and as he speaks there is wonder and a question in his mannerisms. How is it that today he still feels unlovable? The deep sadness and the sense of a young child surround John, who is at least six feet tall and over 190 pounds.

The younger in an extended family that honored only the oldest child, Julia has been unable to gain a centered sense of self or to have confidence in herself. She deeply feels the pain of being, as she says, "not normal." I asked her what was happening within herself that required drugs (Lamb, 2010, p. 142).

Julia: It feels like I don't matter. I don't have anything worthwhile to contribute or say to anybody. Nothing I say makes a difference or nobody really wants to hear what I have to say. Yeah, just sort of I don't matter to anyone or anything or just shuffle me off out of the way.

Ruth: Did those feelings make it easier to turn to an addiction or drugs or alcohol? Did those feelings have any connection with that behavior?

Julia: I think so. Yeah. Trying to fill empty feelings,

emptiness. Or...a sense of low. Yeah, because I guess there's a loneliness with that, too. And stress because I'm not myself. I'm fragmented and things aren't right within myself, so I have to comfort myself or drown out my feelings because my feelings are trying to tell me that something's wrong. Because all the feelings and instincts and stuff...You know, this isn't the right way to live. So I have to shut it down because I don't know how to deal with it.

Ruth: So you shut it down.

Julia: I don't have any tools to fix myself.

Ruth: Your tool became the drugs and alcohol?

Julia: Yeah, just sort of...It's too painful, so I needed to use to take the pain away.

Julia: It's been a long time with the negative feelings.

Ruth: Was there a benefit from those negative feelings, do you think? Some way they served you?

Julia: Yeah, in some ways they served. Maybe they protected me or something, I don't know.

Ruth: So, they protected you. That's important. Do you have any idea how those negative feelings protected you?

Julia: Maybe if I was telling myself all of these negative things, then I was expecting that everyone else was thinking it so I'd be the first one to tell myself. And then if everyone else told me it wouldn't be so hard.

Soon the story becomes untenable as Julia increases her drug use until she is listening to the negative voice, almost totally bound to her bedroom and completely isolated. Before long this negativity overwhelmed her, and her cells. She is diagnosed with Multiple Sclerosis, and her emotional state is now considered bipolar.

Emil portrays more closely the notion of the sorrowful child as the primary subpersonality focus (Lamb, 2010, pp. 136– 137). Emil describes a more unconscious process of separation from self, most likely compounded by many unremembered assaults on his sensitive child nature. He shows me his addiction chart and downplays many sorrowful occasions; however, for the first time in his life he shares what he calls his greatest heart rendering grief.

> Emil: This is my addictions chart. So it is the nature of what I was doing to a timeline of what was actually going on in my life. But at this point, when it came up, when I started doing drugs, there wasn't really anything going on in my life. There's been a lot of grief. There have been a lot of losses throughout my life.
>
> Ruth: There have been losses in your life.
>
> Emil: Oh yeah, by all means. Where in fact, this was the biggest one that's played on my life for quite some time and I've never talked about it until I came into treatment sixteen years later.
>
> Ruth: Never talked about the biggest trauma?
>
> Emil: I didn't, I couldn't....I was twenty. She would be eighteen at the time. She was pregnant, she wasn't ready for a baby and she got an abortion. After some time I married her, had one child, and then divorced her much later.

Ruth: Everything built up?

Emil: Oh, it really does. It absolutely does. It was overwhelming. I'd never dealt with it in the past. I didn't want any part of the abortion. In fact, I remember sitting there beside her on the bed crying and asking her not to go through with it. There was nothing I could do...Like I say, a month ago I wouldn't even have been able to talk about it. I'd think about it and I'd cry.

For sixteen years, the heartache of his girlfriend's abortion of their fetus weighed on him and brought tears to his eyes each time he reflected on it. He had never shared his pain and inner shame; added to childhood family tensions he never dealt with, this led to his marital failure. For a time, he was able to use drugs to suppress this and other life stresses, as well as his father's sudden death. He could pretend all was well, but deep inside, his decision closed his heart.

Emil's sadness over many occasions both here and in his country of origin left him isolated and feeling detached—drugs brought the release. Grief and sadness expressed during the treatment program brought him awareness and relief.

The dyad here swings between feeling unlovable and sorrowful; either mood or emotional-vital state can drive the addiction. However, it is common for the swing to sadness to sink into depression—a common diagnosis in our study. Amber, Julia, and Emil were able to articulate their unlovability, as did John. It is as if the lower emotional-vital holds the belief in its clutch and releases the toxic awareness at regular intervals to self-punish and inevitably shroud the soul-consciousness. Solace then comes from outside in the form of the addictive substance.

Addict versus divine-child

The voice of the addict is capable of overriding all

restraint—that is, all but a deeper spiritual longing and sublimated faith. Emil describes in his own words (Lamb, 2010, p. 152):

> Emil: My heart was telling me that I wasn't happy. Honestly, every time I got high I told myself that it was the last time. Each time I told myself it was the last time.
>
> Ruth: How come it wasn't?
>
> Emil: It was the drugs and what they did. I'm reflecting back on that day I gave everything up. It was my heart that told me to do that.

Not only Emil, but also Paul expressed the driven nature of desire for the substances they were using.

> Paul: When I came into the programs I was frightened. Like I say, I was emotionally destroyed and I...I let God back into my life. I always believed in God. Literally, like I say, I bopped around in AA for almost a year and it wasn't the alcohol that was taking me out. I could go without alcohol but I had a really hard time dealing with cocaine. I'd get thirty days, sixty days and crash. That compulsion would just come over me and nothing else mattered. I would get thirty days in and go, "Oh, this is a milestone. I'd better go get some cocaine" and celebrate. That this insane thinking with my addictions.
>
> Ruth: You called that insane thinking.
>
> Paul: When I came in here for treatment, I had 122 days of sobriety and when the Friday night before the Sunday I thought "Oh, I better go out and have one more yeehaw" and they almost kicked me out of here but I was honest with them and I'm glad I was. I was only scheduled to be phase 2, but they put me

back into scheduling in phase 1 and I am so thankful for that because I wanted, I needed what they had to offer me. And I saw the difference with the other people that were in my group and they fought it and they ignored it and I just realized that's the addict. And I don't want that.

Crucial perhaps to Paul's ongoing successful recovery is that he was able to gain some distance, open to his witnessing aspect, and name the 'addict'. Owen, even as young as 20, has a good grasp mentally of what he is up against.

Owen: You know the action that you um...that you're doing. You know the thing that you do um in order to get it. Um, the will of my...the addict within me and the will of my...the addict will do anything to get high. To get out of my head and like you know its... its...it comes to a point where you lean on it so much and the things only get worse and only exacerbate the problem. I mean he'll never...he'll never, I mean...this addict, he may stop eating for awhile. I say eating into my soul or feeding on my soul you know. The addict eats away at my soul.

The 'addict' seduces so successfully—it takes over, it controls, it offers sly and sneaky suggestions, and it likes to present its habitual thought forms as if they are naturally right for action. For many, listening and succumbing takes them to a place of bottoming out, or as several clients mentioned, being done. Being done refers to borderline toxicity, to knowing death may be near, and in some cases, to actively seeking an end to this 'artificial insanity' (Lamb, 2010, p. 152).

Each client was asked what brought them into treatment. Responses often provided insight into how the addict subpersonality entices the desire-nature, and amazingly, how the deeper spiritual core—the soul-centered essence—can sneak through. The spiritual core thus provides just the synchronicity required to support faith and activate a healing strategy: the Divine child comes forth. We start with Paul who is clean and who recently telephoned to say he has become an addiction treatment counsellor (Lamb, 2010, pp. 107-117).

Ruth: What brought you into treatment?

Paul: I became a cocaine user when I was 22, and at 49 I'd experimented with crack cocaine for almost 27 years. I was very lucky to be alive. I was done. You're sitting there with half an ounce of cocaine and a bottle of whisky and it's four in the morning and you're looking out and I've actually smoked myself sober, where I'm asking God why has it taken me so long to realize that I can't take care of this problem. I realized that if I kept up the way I was living my life, I was going to die. I was spiritually bankrupt. I had ruined so many relationships. Emotionally I was a mess. Health-wise, just about destroyed, borderline toxic. The only thing I did do in my recovery is I always ate. I ate and drank lots of water and that's a testimony that I'm still alive today. I truly believe that.

Paul woke up the next morning and prayed to be helped; this time, he says, he really meant it. Within minutes of leaving his apartment he met the father of a friend whom he had not seen for years, and this father was a member of AA. Paul asked him for information; it took one more week of cocaine and alcohol, but the end was near. He followed up, joined AA, and sought admission to the treatment centre.

In another moment, Emil shared what finally brought him to treatment.

Ruth: What brought you into treatment now?

> Emil: Like, my poison? What I was doing? I guess I knew that enough was enough. I'd known for a long time that enough was enough. What had happened was I went on a binge... Like, I was working all at the same time. And I'd come off a binge of two or three days in and I went to work on the Monday. My boss caught me. I woke up that Monday morning and I said, "enough is enough" and I knelt by my bed and I started praying, "Let me know what I need to do." No more than a half an hour after I got to work, my boss said he needed to talk to me. So I laid it all out on the table for him. I told him exactly what I was doing. How long I'd been doing it for. What I wanted to do for myself. And that whole thing took six hours. We talked for six hours. He stood up and he said, "Okay, print out exactly your plan, send out the email to everybody you're on stress leave. Go do what you want to do. Go do what you think is best for you." That afternoon I came home, I was able to call a counselor.

Emil's prayer was answered that morning after several years of addictive behavior, the boss chose that very morning to confront Emil.

Amber's story was similar. I asked her, "What brought you into treatment at this time, Amber?" and she replied:

> Basically, I couldn't deal with my emotions and my feelings anymore. And I've always resorted to alcohol and drugs in my whole life. And because I'm in my 40s I guess that thing called "progression" has happened, that I just learned about here. It's like where you saturate your body and damage your neurotransmitters...Like, you're basically done. If I were to do it more, I would get more adverse affects as opposed to the affects that I've always gotten. So, basically, it was more unpleasurable than pleasurable.

Amber had reached a place of 'no gain'; Luke increased his cocaine dosage until he thought he was having a heart attack.

> Luke: Yeah. And it's quite a bit. So that would be... one, two, three....That would be a half a gram, three grams, so that's what....six times more.

> Ruth: Did it just stop working? Is that why you did so much?

> Luke: I don't know. We just started doing more and more. Yeah. It just didn't stop, right? It kept going. I thought I was going to die. Yeah. I felt like I was having an overdose. I thought I was going to pass out. I felt like I was going to pass out. And it was like an extreme high anxiety and my heart wouldn't stop pounding. Then even a few days later, it would still do the same thing, even the next week. It just happened all of a sudden...I went from having a good time, thinking we're having a good time to that point, to thinking I was going to die.

Looking out his window one night around that time, Luke saw a full moon—to his culture this is an important moment. He prayed for assistance. Somehow he activated his supports, withdrew from an abusive alcoholic mother who lived with him, and entered treatment.
Samuel shared:

> Samuel: I'm just tired of keeping going the way I've been going. Drugs are no answer.

> Ruth: How come they're not the answer?

> Samuel: Nothing really good ever came of them. I mean, with me, broke all of the time. It caused problems in my marriage. In general, it was havoc throughout my whole life. I mean, it's put me in

jail and I really blame a lot of this stuff on him [his father]and then after a while, it's me, you know? I've been trying to get ready for years and don't know how. I've tried lots of things—praying, I've tried breathing, I've tried just lots of stuff. I've just never gotten counseling. I've never talked about it. The first time I've ever talked about it was in groups here. I didn't even talk about it in front of my sister when we had family day, just the other day. So it's pretty...Like, she knows what went on. She's not stupid. She lived through it too, but she chose not to do drugs. She got, I guess, help from where she worked and I just kept doing drugs. That was my help.

Ruth: And now that doesn't work?

Samuel: Well, no. Now it's addiction, full-blown addiction. It does nothing except make me paranoid and I get psychotic. Not all the time I get psychosis but there's those times that yeah, if I use enough throughout the day I will...Shoot, actually psychosis starts right away, right now.

Samuel hears voices; he knows they are not him but they are present with him much of the time. Interestingly, Samuel felt Jesus's presence with him during his first treatment. He somehow felt the power of Jesus's robe and spoke later of how he pictures the robe and its colors near him when he is anxious. He uses this initial image as a strategy to sustain him through stressful times.

Andy hit bottom and he knows it.

Ruth: You kept seeking recovery, a little bit, even on your own in the recovery house?

Andy: Well, first of all, I was really sick of the drugs.

I was sick of just the feeling that I would get from them. Well, they worked, but they didn't work in the same sense as when I really first started using, before it was more of a social kind of fun thing. And by the end, there's no social aspect of it. There's no fun in it. Before I would do them, I would tell myself, "Okay, I don't want to do them." Like, I'll go get some food and go this or that. And before you knew it, I'm doing the drugs again and once they're gone, I'm feeling ten times worse than before. It's just like a vicious cycle.

Ruth: So you started to notice the vicious cycle.

Andy: Yeah, worse and worse and worse. From what I've heard from other people, too, that is pretty common. It grabs hold of you and then you just spiral down. And that's why in recovery people talk about their bottoms because you spiral down until you hit the bottom whether it's a financial bottom, a physical bottom or an emotional bottom, which they all are very, very deep and hurtful, but they all are different, too, in the same sense. They have a different affect on me and my body.

Ruth: So there's some bottom that registers.

Andy: Yeah, yeah. Something has clicked and goes, "What am I doing?" For the majority of the people that I have met, they have reached a bottom and that's why they've made the conscious choice to seek help. And everybody is different. For some people they might have to go ten feet down. Or some people might just have to go two feet down. So...

Ruth: How did you know you'd hit your bottom? What

kind of signs were there in your life?

Andy: In my life...Well, I lost my apartment. I had to move in with my cousin. I lost my job. I had to go back to my old job. There were a number of factors, I guess, myself hitting the bottom, myself just being really sick and tired of feeling ashamed and guilty and disappointing people as well as myself. That's what really kind of changed me.

Ruth: Inside you it changed?

Andy: Inside me, yes. Like, inside my heart and inside my mind.

Andy could articulate that his heart had opened. He felt compassion for the first time for himself, his struggles, and the individuals who had suffered because of his breaking and entering crime behaviors. He had always blamed himself and listened to the addict-voice that promised solace, but he was clear that drugs no longer kept their promise. However, his four friends who were like brothers to him (he grew up with them and saw them every day) were addicts. He knew this would be a problem, and he also knew he had changed inside; nevertheless, once he was out of the centre he did return to drugs. Within three months he had placed himself back in treatment. Let us hope he has gained enough ego strength, enough heart-opening self-love, and enough cognitive tools to succeed.

Owen's bottoming out hit a new low as he tightened the belt around his neck.

So at some point the consequences became too much for me to bear, just constant feelings of...I really did want to die. I didn't want to take my life so much and I, I, I would go through certain um like I would put the belt around my neck, but never, you know, try to choke the life out of myself. Just...and but I was inching closer and closer and I felt ...uh I felt that my life was in danger. I was endangering myself and I was endangering other people. You know I didn't...I didn't know um if I would...when I broke into someone's car if the owner would come up behind me. What would I do then? Obviously I would fight them. I didn't want to go to jail...I was so used to stealing from my family without...with very little consequences.

The addict was in for self-destruction; it was Owen's insight and awareness that overcame the false desire to end his life. Time and time again Owen showed insight—cognitive awareness of his state and behaviors. He could save his life from the belt, but he could not end the addiction at the time of the research.

John speaks of the ultimate despair.

John: There was a time at the recovery house where I made a decision that I didn't want to live and I took some pills. Not enough to kill me but...I did know in my heart that if I had enough, I would have done it. I hit bottom when I was there. When I started feeling again, it was horrible.

Ruth: So when the drugs wore off, you started having your normal feelings?

John: Yeah, that was the worst.

Ruth: And you had no tools?

John: There's nothing. No. There was nothing that was going to help me because my brain chemistry would have...it was so out of balance from all the drugs. The depletion of all the chemicals I needed to feel okay. That topped with the loss. Like, coming to after six months and then looking at the destruction. It's as much as a feeling of despair as I think one could... being out on the middle of the ocean hoping a ship comes by. The feelings of despair, I've never been out on the middle of the ocean but I know of despair.

The addict took John to despair and to enough pills to almost succeed in suicide; however, as soon as he awoke in the hospital, he called and asked to return to the study and to his healing sessions. On the phone he said, "I want to find my faith again". As far as we know at this time, John succeeded. He did as he noted: He found his faith and he turned his stubborn side into an ally.

With Jasper, the early trauma, family history of drug use, use of multiple drugs, and deep personalized ambivalence brought challenges:

Jasper: Well, addiction takes over. So by that time you may even want to quit. You may go years telling yourself that you're going to quit and then you're able to stop thinking about it for a couple of weeks or a month and then you really want to quit. You realize it's destroying your life but you don't really know how to do anything else, so you just continue. And a lot of people will say they stop getting high. They got a buzz but they didn't get the high they originally got. It just maintained. So for a long time, usually they say until you have this drastic bottom or you hit the point where you finally say "things can't get any worse than this, I might as well try going without." And that's different for different people.

Ruth: Did you hit what you'd call a bottom?

Jasper: Yes, several times. I tried to kill myself several times and the last time was a few weeks ago. I spent a month in the hospital. They committed me and I was able to detox in there. And I got a bit of a clearer head. I wasn't using and I thought maybe I can do it.

Ruth: So you haven't used since June?

Jasper: I was using while I was in the hospital, but only marijuana, I hadn't drank, I hadn't used cocaine. And I thought marijuana was the one thing I wouldn't have to give up. Everything else was dangerous, but marijuana wasn't, is what I used to think. So when I got out, I went to AA and I didn't think marijuana was opposed or something that would be an issue with AA because it's drinking only, right? But I began to realize from a lot of the people that go to AA and from the actual AA program that it has to be complete abstinence from all mood altering drugs. So gradually I quit that too.

After many years of drug use and repeated suicide attempts, Jasper said he had hit the 'drastic bottom'.

'Hitting bottom' expresses itself in numerous ways; here, participant-clients shared the salient features of this most uncomfortable and frightening personal experience. From this uncomfortable place, risking everything is not far.

John: Yeah, I worked. I mean, I've worked…I mean, in the last eight years I've probably done better…for the most part been clean except for this last time I lost everything in six months. Home, job, I had a business, relationships, my child is with his mother. I mean, I just…basically I left. I built up a life and I walked away from it.

Ruth: Because of the drug or just because you wanted to?

John: The drugs. I chose…I basically gave up.

Ruth: Gave up to the drug you mean?

John: My life.

Ruth: For the drug.

John: Yeah. Yeah, it's pretty powerful. It was a big decision, I'll tell you that.

Ruth: Was it a decision?

John: At some point it was, yeah. At some point I decided that life...I convinced myself that life wasn't worth it and there was no other way to... Then I couldn't stop so I didn't even try. I had lots of money so I just used every day. I completely shut myself off from anybody that I'd known before in recovery.

Ruth: What ended that shut-off and just drugging?

John: Because...well, a lot of things accumulated. Like, I was going to jail, committing crimes. I was on the street. I was going to hospitals. I had infections...I was running from the cops and...one day I started on the detox and then I went to detox three times. Then the last time there was just...I guess I didn't have anything left in me. I couldn't fight anymore. I gave up because the reality was that I was going to go to jail because I was doing crimes all over the place. The police already knew me. I was homeless. Overly unhealthy. I was probably 70 pounds lighter than I am now. I had infections. Suicidal. You name it. There wasn't anywhere to go.

Ruth: Nowhere to go.

John: No. Except jail, which I knew that was going to happen. (Lamb, 2010, p. 158).

One way or another, the addict as subpersonality—as a constellated crystallized energy form and consciousness—imprisons individuals, as it imprisoned all of our clients. Some were able to resurrect their faith, hope, and innermost knowing, and when they were at their most hopeless, they 'called' on the greater Divine. When listening to these clients, it felt to me as if the young, innocent, child-like Divine stepped forth as rescuer, and while embracing the adult-self, sent out the 'call'.

From the emotional-vital perspective (as noted above) the more emotional and cognitive explanations are shared. As they formulate in subpersonalities, the force, energy, and crystallized consciousness take on a power that reinforces the fractured ego state and therefore keeps the personality in degrees of confusion and chaos. This alone presents a great challenge to healing processes and treatment programs, but there is even more when we examine Sri Aurobindo's teachings.

The subpersonalities acting as a subterfuge agents are vulnerable to subliminal forces, especially from the subconscient. They can be empowered by a warped lower or middle emotional-vital desire-nature that, for example, drives self-blame: the wounded child in self-blame. There is another wounded child in a constellation of consciousness that calls for self-solace, hence the drugs and all the false promises they elicit.

The following subpersonalities were selected following a reanalysis of the research data: victim-child versus abuser-child; responsible-child versus rebel-child; carefree-child versus fearful-child; unlovable-child versus sorrowful-child; and addict versus the Divine-child. These pairs show the archetypal forces pervading each subpersonality: addict-essence versus soul- presence. Of course, there are other crystallized energies that impact. The bully-child can come under the abuser-child; the angry-child can come under the fearful-child; the silent-child can come under the victim-child; and the Divine-child could be termed soul-presence, an essence of spiritual force. Each aspect, if energized enough, becomes a distinct but incoherent personality capable of stepping forth. Usually, through some desire nature or rajastic quality, the aspect takes a stand and pushes aside the now-fractured centralizing egoic structure.

With the subpersonality is the shadow of a potential light, or the lesson and the potential gift. In understanding and healing the rift created by the fractured ego, the personality can centralize and gain stability. Within each subpersonality there is a hidden aspect of light and a shadow of darkness: consciousness and energy are there, as are information, energy, and power for better or for worse. Choice becomes the master card, complex multidimensional choice—choice that comes from numerous angles and can change in an instant, depending who or what is empowered.

Complex links are interwoven among the outer being nature, the inner being, the innermost being, and the environment. Sri Aurobindo tells us: "Nature being a complex unity and not a collection of unrelated phenomena, there can be no unbridgeable gulf between the material existence and this vital or desire-world" (Ghose, 1996, p. 434). So not only the personal environment needs to be considered but also the relational environment, the community and cultural environment, the media environment, and the multifaceted political environment, to mention some key mediators and drivers of the desire-nature. We return to these environmental mediators in chapter ten under the discussion of thought-forms.

The personality directed by the split-off subpersonalities, the false-personality creates porous boundaries because the individual does not have a clear sense of self—and these porous boundaries leave openings for desire-nature. In effect, porous boundaries have openings for emotional or feeling-toned influences from the many voices held in each subpersonailty, the voice of the aspect that has the focus, and multiple voices from the subconscient. The personalized voices are usually habitual, have gained power over time, and have created considerable consciousness-based habit-pattern grooves within the outer and inner being. Some voices are mechanical and rote, others flare up once triggered by inner or outer circumstances, and others are quite awake and aware and are capable of manipulating through enthusiasm or feeling-driven rationalizations.

In terms of the research clients, addiction brought physical craving as a mechanical desire that impacted, and was often initiated by the feeling emotional-vital lower nature. The stories behind the wounds, while based in a somewhat higher aspect of the vital, interacted with the physical craving and many times provided fuel for the fire that enabled rationalization for the phone call to the dealer and another trip to self-solace—and, when this did not work, often to despair.

There is also a vulnerability to forces within the environment: from people, family, cohort groups, and individuals with a vested interest in clients remaining vulnerable, split, and tied to their wounded nature. These aspects are discussed under the mental body consciousness in chapter ten. Next, we examine the subliminal from the context of the subconscient lower realm of emotional-vital—the realm where wars are created.

9

WAR ZONE CONSCIOUSNESS

Other forces from the subliminal are less well understood but not unknown. Sri Aurobindo remarks:

> Falsehood...is created by an Asuric power which intervenes in this creation and is not only separated from the Truth and therefore limited in knowledge and open to error, but is in revolt against the Truth or in the habit of seizing the Truth only to pervert it. This Power, in the dark Asuric Shakti or Rakshasic Maya, puts forward its own perverted consciousness as true knowledge and its wilful distortions or reversals of the Truth as the verity of things. It is the powers and personalities of this perverted and perverting consciousness that we call hostile beings, hostile forces. (Ghose, 2000a, p. 381).

Our struggle to remain surface—material glued to empiricism, to our beliefs that what we see is all there is— blinds so many to the grander story of humanities capacity for wisdom. He continues:

> The hostile forces exist and have been known to yogic experience ever since the days of the Veda and Zoroaster in Asia (and the mysteries of Egypt and the cabbala) and in Europe also from old times. These things, of course, cannot be felt or known so long as one lives in the ordinary mind and its ideas and perceptions; for there are only two categories of influence recognizable, the ideas and feelings and actions of oneself and others and the play of environment and physical forces. But once one begins to get the inner view of things, it is different (p. 393).

Steeped in desire-based feeling, these forces place power and pressures on individuals, accurately aiming at the areas of weaknesses—splits in wholeness.
Sri Aurobindo tells us:

> It is not surprising that they [hostile forces] should be powerful in a world of ignorance for they have only to persuade people to follow the established bent of their lower nature, while the Divine calls always for a change in nature...But their temporary success does not bind the future. (Ghose, 2000a, p. 398).

Life presents us with challenges and choices, particularly (as great literature assures us) when we seek more coherence, light, purity, clarity, and higher truths. Sri Aurobindo states that the dialectic of challenge and choice is the process of the Golden Law: Each step taken on the upward evolutionary path brings, quite without our conscious permission, a step downward onto the involutionary path. Integral yoga teachings encourage individuals to find the positive in the negative and overcome the adversity by bringing the light of the highest consciousness attainable to the issue (Ghose, 1996, 2000c).

The teachings assure us, reinforcing the notion repeatedly, that the law of descent is commensurate with the law of ascent. They also caution us to not push beyond our ability to hold the light, not to force ourselves to go beyond what we have the consciousness ability to cope with, and especially not to descend to places we are not naturally ready to address. This caution is particularly poignant and a necessary wisdom for all who work with others therapeutically.

Despite the significant fear and superstition surrounding consciousness and energies not understood over time, and the stigma toward those who 'see' and 'know', there have nonetheless been those who with wisdom 'see' and 'know' in cultures throughout time—they are usually honored by the culture. True wisdom for these people often came with deep *tapasaya*. Each of us, if we look, has our own heaven and our own hell, and wisdom teachings assure us that none can reach heaven without passing through hell.

Hell, in this context, is becoming consciously aware of the key problems and challenges cycling in one's life. The problems and challenges as they cycle through are invitations to awaken, to ascend or evolve to the next level; the push or pressure from the soul presents itself in myriad forms of stumbling, falls, and sufferings. Consciousness is needed again and again as disorders resurface in different guises, each time requiring light, calm, hope, faith, wisdom, as well as aspiration, rejection, and surrender to the wiser knowing and higher calling. We are reminded in these teachings to let the future draw us and to make the superconscient the true foundation—not the wounds of the past. Nevertheless, we must be prepared for the dual movement: each step upward complemented by a step downward.

Although theoretical descriptions are important, examples of processes that impact us all in differing degrees bring the teachings forward, grounding them in actual life experiences. Integral yoga teachings remind us that real understanding comes once knowledge is embodied: stories of actual experiences open portals to embodiment (Sri Aurobindo, see Ghose, 2000c). Here, the emotional-vital view of subpersonalities as depicted in the clients from my research (Lamb, 2010). is used to provide actual examples of experiential processes designed to sustain healing.

The new look at the research asks a question: Is it possible that the subpersonality splits provided a portal for adverse forces from the clients' subconscients and the greater subliminal? Once the fractured ego was flooded with a wide variety of trauma or temptations, and the subpersonalities empowered, it was not long before more than the individual's own weaknesses seduced and clouded the mind and higher vital. Tamas and a variety of self-depreciating schemas are empowered, including despondency, and 'off to the races we go' as Paul noted when he was overtaken by the addict subpersonality (Lamb, 2010).

Sri Aurobindo's teachings (Ghose, 2000c) are clear that there can be adverse forces behind self-destructive suggestions. These forces solicit a wrong understanding, and these subtle suggestions press on already established weaknesses: the collapse begins, or conversely, the battle. This 'war zone consciousness' is not an unusual state of being for those who wish to understand and integrate, or even overcome, an activated and destructive subpersonality force of energy (or any other empowered negative force of consciousness.)

Meaningful change can be difficult—particularly for clients with an addiction, and especially if they have had childhoods that did not support and sustain a normal enough, stable, and caring environment. The fragile ego is easily flooded by the emotional-vital and physical as well as the mental outer and inner being subliminal and subconscient forces. Some forces aim to protect the healing process, and others to detract.

Specifically in this case, we examine the forces that detract—that is, that simply will not allow a 'new me' to evolve. This fragile time of change following decisions to heal holds potential, but is ripe for sabotage. It is best to be prepared and even have some understanding of the complexities involved in an integral process of change. The following section presents additional research results, abridged. In each case client and practitioner established a relationship that is co-creative and designed to support the clients where they are in the moment while reinforcing the healing power of consciousness in all its manifestations (Lamb, 2010).

Self-sabotage and old-me-versus-new-me battles occur throughout the recovery process, and were present in the interviews and shared in the healing sessions. This self-sabotage process is a war and it is paradoxically challenging given it includes so many levels of being. For clients who are still finding their worthiness and stabilizing their ego-sense related to who they can become when clean and sober, challenges are formidable. There is much yet to be learned. Once eyes are open and the tremendous complexity of our human condition is acknowledged, a more sophisticated learning adventure can formally begin.

The lower astral (subcontient) world that is known for its massive, frequency-dimensional capability showed itself in language such as heavy energy, dark energy, negative energy, cords, and a range of intrusive energies. Practitioners have their own wording based on their particular lens of high-sense perception, with some practitioners more kinesthetic and others more clairvoyant. All are working with a refined intuitive sense developed from years of detailed healing work and natural self-development practice.

In each case there is a uniqueness in how astral influences impacted these clients. The practitioners, while challenged, showed advanced awareness on how to safely practice healing with such vulnerable clients, and how to keep safe as a practitioner with forces of consciousness that have been documented in many cultures throughout time, yet are new to the paradigmatically changing model of addiction recovery within the research study (Lamb, 2010).

Safely unstacking repressed, entangled, corded, imploded energy held tightly for reasons of self-protection (a wise survival strategy that turned ultimately destructive) is an advanced practice in the newly emerging healthcare profession of biofield therapy. Releasing *crystallized* energy-consciousness-force, held in forms that articulate with anger, rage, grief, shame, or guilt, requires an ability to not only purge and clear subtle emotion- powered material, but also to titer the amount and force of the release and appropriately disperse or transform the subtle packaged matter. Moreover, this release and clearing must make some sense to the client not only experientially, but also cognitively; without at least some rudimentary understanding, the human energy field will not hold a re-patterning and the same vibratory resonating forces can return. In addition, strategically, these changes must fit within the now-forming sense of self that is organizing around evolutionary tapasya processes: the commitment to change, to create and follow another ideal in life.

For a moment though let's take a look at Aliva's comments about how she felt following a counseling session she attended prior to entering the treatment centre. Aliva's case provides an example of what can happen after a counseling session when etheric forces are activated. (She was attempting to come off drugs and had sought counseling support). In her words:

> I was having more nightmares. I was starting to have flashbacks and I had to use more drugs and it was really obvious to me that drugs weren't going to help. So I thought I would just get some psychiatric help. There was one woman I really clicked with but the minute I left her office I phoned my dealer because I thought I had all this swirly stuff moving inside me.

The question is how to clear or purify and then dynamically stabilize a human energy field immersed in an evolutionary healing-learning process; this task is complicated by the knowledge that the involutionary and evolutionary processes work in tandem. One step forward in purification brings its clarity and lessons and new visions of potential; nevertheless, it also calls us to the next task. Fear of that next task may lead the client back to the lower, involved, and masked forces capable of destroying progress. Clients underwent this two-way battle: truly a war zone.

The initial clearing and releasing of entangled energy forces and forms required client participation to be effective— that is, to provide experiences that often triggered not only memories of the trauma experienced and the emotions and feelings repressed, but also memories and perceptions of seeing, hearing, and knowing related to the event. Often, the clients were very engaged and able to assist in powerful releases of encapsulated toxic crystallized energy. Using their heightened sense perception they acknowledged the forms and the emotions held by the forms taken by the lower energy-consciousness—this recognition brought client self-empowerment. They knew they did not want to be manipulated by forms that were not of their true nature.

Amber provided an example of the entranced state:

Amber: I can't remember really what happened but I just went into that trance and I picked my face so bad for the first time that I couldn't actually go out of my house for like a week. I didn't go to work. I didn't leave. I had to get aloe vera plants, and hydrogen peroxide and heal. And now I have a whole routine of picking and healing which is pretty pathetic. Do you understand that?

Ruth: I hear you. What is it you are achieving by picking? Use your high sense perception, your intuition here. What is it achieving?

Amber: It's almost externalizing how ugly I feel on the inside and making it on the outside. So I just don't want to look okay because I am not.

Ruth: When you check inside Amber, can you find a place that feels okay?

Amber: [places her hand on her abdomen and above

her heart] It takes a lot of concentration, but I am learning.

The subliminal subconscious relates to the inner being processes and the manner in which crystallized energy is configured within the human energy field, whether in tissues, between tissues, or in the auric field off the body. Using high sense perception, practitioners and clients alike were able to feel, see, or hear the vibratory resonance from intrusive energy forces. (Again, individuals had their own unique access abilities). A crucial rule of practice in this study was that only what is ready to be cleared is to be cleared—to the best of the practitioner's ability working alongside the client, only what is ready (however small or big) is invited to clear. This readiness factor is a matter of practitioner skillset and internal maturity, as a practitioner must assess both practitioner and client readiness, and the readiness of the client's energy- consciousness-force.

In seven healing treatment appointments, only so much re-patterning could realistically stabilize and integrate, as each step forward brought a counter-attack. Managing this case process, building self-confidence in the client, forging new energetic patterns in the human energy field, and empowering the evolutionary tapasya's inner and outer processes became a healing-learning journey for both client and practitioner. However, it was the practitioner's responsibility to ensure that the multidimensional process sustained the healing choice factors for the client. The clients then had to make the choices— this was their freedom, now that they had at least a rudimentary understanding of the choice and the new potential futures available to them. Accessing and maintaining a new possibility (one of healing and learning) requires personal work, effort, access to soul forces and Grace—or a Divine or Gnostic trust in a greater power—as well as a constant aspiring focus, a vigilant ability to reject detracting forces, and a willingness to surrender to the notion that a new future is indeed possible.

Clients arrived with some degree of aspiration that needed to be reinforced, and they did not understand the complexities involved when a multidimensional rejection of detracting forces responds. The 'no' to drugs, the emotion-management taught by counselors in the treatment facility, and the cognitive strategies based on mental models were extremely helpful, but were not enough unto themselves. To compliment this excellent facility treatment program, clients were guided to other-dimensional healing. The subtle inner being aspect underlying the outer behaviors required attention to allow deepening and assist in sustaining choices for a new and healthier life.

As clients dialogued and met in group, some of the energetic debris held by negative and painful emotions cleared— a superficial clearing that allowed for greater clarity and supported positive decision-making. However, the deeper, more resistant, toxic crystallized energy required intentional dyadic healing processes. This process required practitioner awareness of the need for human energy field self-protection, concomitant with a personal commitment toward self-growth from a healing- learning perspective, and an always reaffirming connection with the Divine source (however the practitioner chose to articulate this belief.)

In summary, the clients' commitment to evolutionary tapasya was crucial. A true intention was required, an aspiration for healing—an ability to reject the early habit-driven urges that would repress and freeze the newly arising feelings and thoughts, combined with a longing to surrender to a regimen of healing that required discipline on their part. Inner technology skills taught and reinforced by practitioners were vital, such as procedures for grounding, centering, and aligning. Clients struggled to remember compassion and the concomitant forgiveness. They strived to focus on self-confession rather than self-blame; this reversal was not easy, as addiction to the lower- order subpersonality schemas that come with self-blame may be a secondary addiction. The human energy field patterning had configured itself to support both addictions—in fact, many addictions—in the form of energetic, physiological, and psychological addictive patterning.

Karen's case (Lamb, 2010, p. 199). offers a useful example. The practitioner reported the following.

> Karen arrives with an intention "to relax into my body and de-stress." She appears to be in an "airy cloud," ungrounded, and her chakras appear to be at a distance from her core...there is a cloudy space between her core and the fogged energies of her chakras. She says she is experiencing, "many moods connected to my addiction to alcohol and drugs." She also states that she has "feelings of loss...too exhausted to cry, feeling frustrated... emotional pain from really missing my child," and is stressed.
>
> Her HEF (human energy field or biofield) central channel alignment moves off to the right. From her 5th chakra her alignment is tilting slightly to her left. Her 1st chakra rotates in a clockwise direction, her 2nd chakra is rotating reverse, and her 3rd chakra rotates reverse, is off center and twisted, deformed and dislocated. Her 4th chakra is rotating clockwise but noticeably small, her 5th chakra is rotating current both directions (mostly clockwise), from her 6th chakra a black strong and extremely powerful cording protrudes and her 7th chakra is small.
>
> I do a Central Channel Alignment to clear some debris (that looks like seaweed swaying), to strengthen and increase the primary energy system in her body, and to connect her chakras to her core. As we progress Karen mentions that she is "experiencing a hard time letting go all of my worries." Eventually her breathing slows, and she surrenders into what appears to be a very peaceful

place. The pulsating black cord from her 6th chakra is holding an incredible amount of energy; it really gets my attention. To do anything with it as a practitioner, would be interference with some, unknown to me right now, universal law. I finish the treatment with good grounding.

Note: This black cord is coming out of her 6th chakra. It is not shown to me whether this cord goes into her spinal column (my sense is that it doesn't.) I couldn't see its ending nor end-attachment in this time. It is pulsating and holds an incredible amount of energy. My sense is that this cord is from another lifetime. How do I know? I just do.

After the treatment Karen says, "I feel so present yet so light...all the heaviness I was experiencing is gone.
I do not feel the frustration or stress, and I am relaxed." Her alignment is straight up to her 5th chakra and from there on is still tilting to her left. Her 4th chakra has expanded.

Comment: My prayer is that: may I show up to receive information in order to assist her healing and at the same time trust and follow my intuition to deepen, create space for consciousness (p. 199).

Another client, John, shared his fear and awareness of astral forces that impact him. He requested two sets of seven Integrative Energy Healing treatments, so we have two practitioner perspectives for his case; it can be seen how important client 'readiness' is and how valuable it is to co- create healing processes with the client.

The first practitioner described the case as follows (Lamb, 2010, pp. 280-288).

John arrives for his first healing session after being in the center 13 days. He has been addicted to crack cocaine for 17 years. He is fidgety and cannot seem to settle in his chair. He finds some intake questions confusing and seems as though he has questions of his own yet can't articulate them. There's is a vacancy in his eyes, just behind that I sense a part of him that can hear and understand what I am saying and that wants to be here and helping himself. His energy field reflects this chaos and his entire body is filled with energetic congestion, in fact I can't locate an area that is clear. His field is prickly, almost electric and a challenge even to touch. He is aware of 'knots' in his stomach, noting, "There's lots of emotion in there." He is also aware of some knee, lower back and joint pain. Although obviously full of concern and emotional discomfort John doesn't even know what 'stress' is. He, however, said his anxiety is high.

John receives an integrative healing treatment detailed in the original text. The practitioner continues her outline of the session.

On completion, John is like a different person. His eyes are clear and bright and he is calm and more grounded. He struggles to find words for this experience but his smile speaks volumes. He shares: "It is so nice. I feel so calm and I am sure you had four or more arms." His stomach feels calmer and the knots are gone. He notes, "I felt like crying when you held my stomach but I didn't." I said that it is fine to cry and we speak about holding on versus letting go. Energetic congestion remains throughout his body but his field is calmer and softer. We worked on the tip of the iceberg today. As he leaves he remarks, "I'll do whatever it takes. I have to. I have to make this work this time."

On his second visit John says, "I have had a tough week but I am learning about reclaiming my personal power." He has energetic congestion in his neck, head and shoulders and the 2nd, 3rd, and 4th chakras with his biofield out from his body 6 inches and very hot, full of static but not as prickly as last week. After clearing and balancing treatments John is able to identify a red and thick cord in his abdomen that needs removing. He identifies that it is to his mom who abandoned him as an infant. He chooses to bring his mom's image forth and dialogues with her. He cries as he speaks softly to her about how much he missed her and needed her and he asks her where she is. When he is complete he chooses to let the unhealthy cord between them dissolve knowing that he can still love her and feel a heart connection. He replaces the area where the cord has been with healing blue light and images of crystals and dolphins. I work with his heart to assist the integration. Then when I move to his head John identifies another energetic cord he describes as "red and orange, it is long...and at the other end is the old John." He dialogues again and dissolves the cord filling the area with 'love'.

At the end of the session John says, "I felt sad letting go but I have to. I feel exhausted and really light. I know I have to force myself to listen to people even if I don't like it." He explains that his foster parents came the other day with their impact letter. "I used my grounding technique while I listened. It helped, just learning all this stuff doesn't help—you have to live it. I am learning that if I can feel it, I can work with it. I am learning that no matter how uncomfortable it feels I can do it. I don't want to run away this time. I feel ready to do it differently this time. I am stubborn, maybe I can use the stubbornness for good."

Through the healing treatments John spoke more about foster homes and about an energetic/psychic type of sensitivity that was likely violated severely though his childhood experiences. He mentions astral travel, fevers, and nightmares as well as panic attacks he experienced as a child. He speaks of a "haunting sensation of a porous substance coming up my throat and filling my mouth"; it paralyzes him with fear.

By the third session John is distraught—he is moving out of the facility to a recovery house tomorrow. He feels suicidal as he does not want the life of an addict again. He is teary in a distant kind of way and does not look directly at me. He looks about to leave but appeared glad to get on the table. His human energy field is almost imperceptible. It is as if it has been drawn back inside him. I note no energetic congestion or any unusual signs notable before in hand scans. Even more than his words of suicide, the change in his human energy field alerts me to the seriousness of the situation.

I began by holding the container of the field off the body, allowing my field to speak to his field encouraging him to 'come back'. I found my grounding and alignment essential here—more so than any other treatment I have done before. I work at not getting drawn into the drama but to meet John where he needs me. I focus on the heart chakra and connecting with John's higher self, asking nonverbally if he can accept the unconditional love and support offered. I work with chakras.

As I reach his heart chakra he shouts "God is testing my will." I ask him very gently what his response to God is and he whispers, "I will never give up." He repeats this over and over, and as he does his field begins to shift and 'return' in small increments. He is much calmer and I ask him to take himself back to a time before the drugs and trauma in his life and to allow his cells to remember. I ask him to breathe his new commitment to never give up into his cells, organs muscles and tissues. He responds with a nod and his field continues to shift as he implements these suggestions. I then ask him to bring healing white light energy in gently through his crown and allow it to move thorough his body pushing out any intrusive energy. I sense several intrusive energies present yet know that he is too fragile to do a conventional extraction. My intention is that this process be gentle as he regains parts of himself and any remaining intrusive energies can be addressed when he is stronger.

John takes time to integrate and when he sits up he remarks, "I am so mean to myself, but I feel better about myself now. I moved some bad stuff out through the tears, mostly unworthiness. Not forgiving myself is the biggest thing—something stops me from forgiving. It feels like a possession to me, something stirs the pot. I was a good kid—I didn't do anything to anyone! I hate that kid [me] even looking back at photos. The abandonment and rejection from my mother is so powerful that I rejected me!" I ask him about the suicidal thoughts. He responds, "I am sorry for saying that to me. It's the part of me that doesn't want to get better." I mentioned how proud I am of him and the work he did today. He cries and says, "That really means something to me, thank you." He adds, "I have seen the destruction of addiction in myself and others. I feel happy that this worked tonight because it's gonna be okay if I am okay. Tonight I felt the presence of God or the Creator. He gave me purpose and direction. I am supposed to help other people."

This was one of the most complex and challenging sessions I have been part of as well as one of the most rewarding. Grounding and alignment were hugely important for the task at hand and the seriousness. I felt quite emotional when I got home. I called the researcher and we discussed how I was feeling and tell her John's words about suicide. She also immediately notified the treatment center and spoke with a counselor there. I did feel a sense of urgency and yet knew that I can only offer the love and support I am able to and that in the end the decision John makes now, or later, is ultimately his. I felt an intense warrior nature come through me in the session, determined to help him fight for his life and at the same time knowing a mothering gentleness was necessary. This session required that I firmly hold the tension of the opposites.

John arrives for session four knowing that we had alerted the treatment center about his discussion regarding suicide and they notified his new recovery house. He vocalizes how upset he is with me for telling the researcher about his suicidal thoughts. There is no aggression or anger, more a sense that I betrayed him. "I never would have told you if I thought you would tell anyone. I am really embarrassed." I offered him my heartfelt apology but told him that I am legally and morally obliged to pass along that type of information, and it had never been my intention to embarrass him. I ask him gently to consider what he might do if a friend he cared for said he or she was considering suicide, whether he would just cross his fingers and hope that wouldn't happen or would he gather all the resources available to find the deserved support. I tell him I think he is worth fighting for. He smiles and we call a truce. I commend him for voicing his feelings to me about my actions. John then starts to cry. Deep wrenching sobs, the kind that words can't offer any solutions to. I support the space we are in energetically. After fifteen minutes he stops crying and climbs on the massage table.

His energy field has expanded only slightly from last week, a bare perceptible 2 inches off the body. Clearing, strengthening, and balancing treatments are used. Again John feels a cord that needs to be released; it is connected to his previous partner of seven years to whom he feels he gives his power and says he is addicted to as well. I assist him with this release while being aware of intrusive energies in his field. He bravely and with some difficulty releases the cord. It is not the time to address the intrusive energies. John looks lighter after the session; he says, "I feel good and I am glad I'm here." We have a long discussion followed by the usual self-care homework.

By the fifth session John has now moved to a senior's house. He talks about his commitment to healing. "I have to take action and do stuff to help others. God will help me change. I can't change but I can take the actions to make a change and hope I will change because of that. I never gave anything or helped anyone before. That's the difference between the other times I tried to stop and now." His human energy field is still very congested, off the body 4 inches. Treatments are directed at clearing stagnant energy and opening a flow between chakra two and four and he asks for integration between his head and his heart. He feels an "opening up in the throat stretching down to my heart." This is especially nice, he explains, because he often has a sensation of concrete being poured here and hardening into a pressure that is very disturbing for him. We also work on liver-clearing, as he is concerned that he has some liver damage. He learns how to support and heal his own liver and agrees to give himself a small treatment each evening. My intuitive sight now sees a small beam of yellow from his solar plexus.

By session six John has started work and has signed up for a three-month program at a hospital for rational emotive therapy. It is three hours a day in a group setting to deal with anger management. He says, "It is considered an intensive program for some, but feels like a downwind for me after all I have been through this year." He speaks for a full hour in this session. He talks about how sensitive he is to other people's feelings. If his adoptive mother was ever angry he felt it was he who caused it. "I always take it personally when others are mad. I feel for them emotionally." He goes on to say how demeaned he felt in childhood and shamed and how he never truly felt loved. "Nothing matters but feeling loved. I didn't get what I needed in childhood. I know I am unlovable and this has taken me to the ends of the earth [suicide]. How many times have I been through this, I know I will be a statistic if I don't pay attention."

His energy field holds a lot of congestion around his head, heart, and solar plexus. His field emanates about 2 feet out from his body, so he did maintain some of our work from last time. We worked on clearing and releasing treatments and then strengthening and balancing for re-patterning his field. John identifies mantras to support him in recovery.

John began the anger-management rational emotive therapy at the hospital, but before the week was out he attempted suicide; he called the treatment center to cancel his healing session because he was in the hospital. A few days later he called me and said he wanted to find his faith again. He asked if he could come back for his remaining healing session or even for more. I agreed but told John he would have a new practitioner, as the seven-week commitment for his first practitioner was complete. He was grateful and readily accepted a new practitioner and another series of treatments, to equal a total of thirteen treatments.

The new practitioner's case notes were as follows.

John presents about ten minutes late, appearing disturbed and somewhat tense, wound up, agitated, not present. He sits down and starts to talk about having to change residences again back to the junior residence given the concerns raised by clients in the senior house since his recent suicide attempt. John says that he was able to state his case but it did not change the outcome.

I sense a strong 'push' from John's energy field while sitting and listening to him. The 'push' has a 'prickly' edge to it. After about twenty minutes I ask John about his experiences with grounding, what he remembers from previous healing sessions, and suggest that we review grounding, centering, and aligning, and accessing spirit while sitting in chairs. Together we reinforce the process.

Overall I sense heaviness throughout his energy field, little flow, edges prickly, well defined on the right and poorly defined on the left. He has more energy to the top of his field and less on the bottom. His left side is more charged than his right side, and he has more energy imploded within than outer. I sense a matrix structure running from his sternum to his diaphragm and heavy energy centered above his left knee. I initiate treatments to clear and smooth his field, to facilitate energy flow, and to remove heavier energies into the ground. Then work on activating a spiral flow to dissipate stagnation in the field. During the brain balance I note fascial unwinding as if an elastic or tight sheet slowly releases after being stretched into a holding pattern. John comments that he can feel the shifts and "It feels good." His energy field responds with some releasing of heavy energy and an improved flow overall.

When we debrief, John comments: "It feels more like raising bread...expanding in my chest and head...that's good, that's okay. When I am feeling depressed I close up...that's what depression is for me." We discuss self-care and his return next week. I can see how the other residents of the senior rehab house could feel unsafe given the intensity of John's field when he is expressing anger or frustration. One test for me is to continually check my grounding, keep my heart open, and boundaries clear to maintain a 'safe' container for John to do his work.

John arrives late and upset for his ninth healing. He has had to address his issues with his former girlfriend, and he had a run-in with a male stranger who is aggressive; he feels rage but did not act on it. While John is relating the events of the past few days he appears overcome at times with emotion, head in hands, rocking back and forth with tears, "My mind is whirling around like a tornado inside my head. I feel like I am possessed, please God, please God."

I sensed his field to be chaotic, very agitated, pushing into my field in waves. I continue to hold space, I ground again, center and align and reground the room with the intention to create a safe container holding John with compassion and detachment from the drama. After about thirty minutes the energy is spent and we ground together. John put his hands over his heart, settles down some more and says it isn't anger, it is frustration and tears of sadness.

Once he is on the table I reassess his energy field: it feels drained at the emotional body and active at the mental body and much calmer overall. There is a strong flow of energy pushing out from an area around his neck and shoulders, a weak flow through his legs, and buzzing static along the surface. His chakras feel absent and in need of filling. I used treatments to clear and purge his field from the heaviness, to strengthen, and to repattern and balance. Most of the treatment time consists of repeated processes of clearing, calming, and repatterning. We debrief, and discuss and reinforce his grounding.

At this point, I discussed John's process and progress with the new practitioner. We were aware that John was likely harboring several intrusive energy forms, as he himself reported and the first practitioner noted. John's transformative healing- learning process was shifting: he was unfolding more awareness and more witness abilities, and as a consequence had moved back into the next level of his unhealed wounds. The pressure to heal maintained its force, and the pull-back to old patterns reactivated this force. This dialectic process was bound to activate intrusive formations of energy that were working to preserve themselves. We discussed a strategy to release the energies that were no longer needed and were detracting from John's healing trajectory.

The practitioner's notes continued:

John arrives for his tenth healing session five minutes late, sits in a chair, head down, slumps, and stares vacuously at the floor. He announces: "I am possessed, I just want to get rid of this feeling." I say, "Okay, let's do it...let's release that feeling." Through the release treatment dialogue, John identifies the energy as "depression" located in the lower part of his abdomen.

As John speaks I sense a dark, very heavy mass between John's 1st and 3rd chakras, its main body lying within the pelvic bowl, with tendrils climbing up the spine and into the back of the heart, other tendrils are noted within the groin and down into the legs. I had no sense that the energy is a disincarnate spirit, when I checked in with the heavy energy it presents itself to be a nonhuman entity attached to and feeding off John's energy system. John and I remain in dialogue. John says he "feels the energy wants to come out through his mouth" and at that point he begins dry heaving, loudly and viscerally.

The process takes some time and remains loud and visceral. I maintain a strong container with the intention of creating a space for John to release this energy, which now forms a molasses-like pudding-like astral energy mass on the floor. I began to energetically invite the earth to receive this astral matter and to call on the Teams of Light and Divine presence to move the energy into the earth for transmutation. When this main process is complete, both John and I go inward again and together track down all the remaining tendrils of attachment. When this completes we go into a purification, protection, guiding light meditation and visualization, one that John will continue to use at home. The scan of his field shows differences throughout but a sense of vulnerability in the areas of clearing. Two other treatments are used to strengthen his field and ensure energy flow throughout. On completion, the vulnerable and stagnant areas are flowing.

John remarks: "I feel a lot better than when I entered, thank you. The heaviness is gone." We discuss self-care and practice his special imagery meditation again. We again practice grounding, centering, aligning, and the need to bring light to those areas where he felt the intrusive formations leave, and the need for him to own those spaces.

I debriefed with the practitioner after this treatment. He did a self-scan ensuring his field was clear, clean, and balanced, and that he had also integrated the meaningful nature of this challenging release treatment. The practitioner's notes continued:

John arrives the following week. This week he wants to soften the fear that resides just under his rib cage and restricts his breathing. He also remarks, "I have been off cigarettes and coffee for six days, my mind is scattered, up and down all week. One minute I am hopeful and the next I want to die." He sits with his arms crossed.

I ask him how old he is. John responds, "five or six. I want something...something in a relationship that I am not getting." I ask, "Can you be with this child, you as a five-year-old child and you as a mid-thirties man? Just be with that aspect of yourself with a soft heart." John starts to sob, tears, head down, heavy emotions release for about ten minutes. I say, "You can have a relationship with your inner child—keep him safe, play, respect him, be in awe and wonder in life—bring this back." John says, "This feels true to me...I can be there for him." I say, "You can be there for yourself, the man, also." John notes, "I sometimes feel this fear in my body, that I won't start the next breath, I won't breathe in, I feel panic and fear that I am going to die. I feel it under my ribs and in my diaphragm...I want to soften, release the fear I feel in this area." I ask, "Is it like you are underwater struggling for life, struggling for air?" John says, "Yeah."

His energy field shows scattered energy, chaotic energy around his head and shoulders and a big farther push of energy off John's head with a weak flow down his legs. Clearing, facilitating, long line flow treatments are selected. I ask John to assist the energy flow of heavy energy down his body and he does so. As I start a brain balance treatment I feel energy pouring through my hands into John's head and a responding movement under my hands from John. I strengthen my grounding and alignment and my breathing pattern deepens to support John in this moment. This intense flow seems to activate John's emotional body aspect of the energetic body, and I note that John's abdomen is filled with worm-like energy that is wrapped around the diaphragm and also filling the space in his abdomen. I invoke Divine assistance, and continue to clear and to disseminate the energy. I then clear his field from head to toe and spend extra time on the rib cage. Following this process John says he can breathe easier. I grounded John and then we move back to the chairs for debriefing and our usual practices of grounding, centering, aligning, and dialogue.

John says, "I feel better now than I did when I came in." I remark, "You are smiling." John says, "Yeah that's more than twice in two weeks. I still feel a little fear off and on...but I feel calm, less scattered."

In our debrief immediately following this session, this experienced practitioner said: "This was a challenging treatment to hold the container, hold my alignment, and continue to return to my heart center as many changes occurred during the treatment session. I bow to John's courage to move through it." Again we ensured that the practitioner's field remained clear. The practitioner's notes continued:

John has two more healing sessions. He learns to ground, center, and align more deeply and to release emotions by washing them down into the earth with his out-breath and to receive clear light with his in-breath. He learns how to address his own frustration, anger, and fear (which continue to confront him) using tools, particularly heart-based focus tools, that nurture grounding, centering, and aligning as well as accessing his sense of God or Divine source. As well as treatments in these last sessions, the focus is on integration through awareness dialogue and reaffirmation of skills and tools for self-care that he has been practicing all along.

John expresses gratitude at closure, "I feel very relaxed, feel good, more together, less scattered."

In our final debrief, the practitioner remarked:

> John can work with his inner awareness, he
> is in his body. He knows that the choices he makes
> matter. We talked about how a plane flying across
> the country needs constant course corrections.
> Adjustments are necessary to keep on the heading.
> John knows that three conscious breaths will bring
> him back to his body, emotions, and mind in present
> time, that he can use the grounding centering and
> aligning and drop into his heart, and from there
> check in with himself.

John was using all his skills, determined to find a
new and transformative way of being in the world. His
battle was rife with dialectically opposing forces; however,
the innermost soul- based promptings seemed to sustain
him even during his worst moments. For example, in his
most recent suicide attempt he did not have enough pills
to succeed and he called for assistance. This led to a
very determined inner push—a force that could not come
forth earlier—to ask for help to do the work it took to free
himself from detracting intrusive forces. The battle then
became even fiercer. By entering another phase of the
transformative healing-learning process, the new added
consciousness force led to the next layer of frustrating
and sometimes overwhelming situations that required his
new skills immediately. He did not always succeed but
he did come for support, and with his practitioner he did
magnificent and challenging work. The slow, multilayered
process held in place by his commitment to heal allowed
the emergence of a new way of being.

John must keep the evolutionary tapasya process
activated, accompanied by greater and greater energy-
consciousness-force applied to ensuring that his aspiration,
rejection, and surrender life-skills continue to grow in
sophistication. At year two of sobriety, John is living in
a recovery house, working, and (as reported by another

client) is staying 'clean' and healthy, and looking good.

For practitioners also, this is not work for the faint of heart. A sophisticated science, multimodal theoretical, and extended clinical biofield educational program is necessary, and even then, as can be seen by the remarks from these experienced practitioners, the healing process is challenging. Practitioners themselves can have an affinity to some of the astral matter and can take on astral forces, as reported on two occasions by practitioners in this research (Lamb, 2010). So, cautionary measures are required and a supportive professional team and environment are advisable.

The emotional-vital holds much power; when the egoic nature is fragile and subpersonalities have been empowered, the evolutionary process presents serious challenges. We examine the physical, subtle physical, nervous system, and cellular responses in a later chapter eleven and twelve.

Remember, there are Powers of Light and Support, to be discussed more as we uncover the layers and manifold aspects of each plane. However, according to Sri Aurobindo's teachings it is the beings of the inner subtle or astral worlds that "try to possess...so that they may enjoy the materialities of physical life without having the burden of the evolution or the process of conversion in which it culminates" (Ghose, 2000, p.386). Understanding this potent perspective allows wisdom and hope, for evolution lies here on the earth. He reminds us:

> The Earth... is an evolutionary world, not at all glorious or harmonious even as a material world (except in certain appearances, but rather most sorrowful, disharmonious, imperfect. Yet in that imperfection is the urge toward a higher and more many-sided perfection (p. 388).

Everyone is challenged—at the highest, we are all One, yet many personalities have greater and lesser degrees of centralization.

The more fractured one is, the more power is received by a false-self, the more porous and numerous are the entry points for vital forces to lead us astray. "What is important to the vital plane is the force or feeling and the form expresses it. A vital being has a characteristic form" (Ghose, 2000, p. 389). However, this vital-being form can vary or mask the true form, or take the place of the true form as consciousness, emotion, and energy congeal into set patterns and vibratory bandwidths.

Understanding how the emotional-vital impacts choice becomes crucial for all change processes. Where the lower vital is driven by instinctual responses, primitive brain coding, and nervous system patterning, the middle vital is susceptible to the egoic desires and subpersonalities in subterfuge. The higher vital connecting the desire-heart and rational mind requires dedicated respect, a power of understanding strong enough to influence choice, and life-force-will for change to occur. With the higher vital in support of the evolutionary process and inner self-development, there can be an ease of awareness when stumblings occur, and a vigilant awakened consciousness alert to adverse circumstances and forces.

In this way, a more coherent, spiritual-warrior consciousness can replace a fear-driven, wounded, and fractured egoic state of being. Subpersonalities can be seen for what they are—split off and wounded aspects of the forming personality, split-off aspects of consciousness that formulated a strategy for survival with the best tools available at the time. These split-off aspects with their own dualities bring strengths and can contribute to a new, mature, centralizing, egoic state of being. As the subpersonalities, defined now to some extent, consciously integrate and empower the centralized ego and lend their gifts to the personality structure, healing is empowered. A 'new-me' personality has greater inner and outer resources. A more forceful upward evolutionary process is initiated, one more equipped to deal with the battle zones sure to follow any true attainment—indeed, ironically, a new battle is a sign of attainment.

The inner and outer vital are intimately intertwined with the inner and outer mental and physical, with the hidden pressures from the soul, and with the often numinous guidance from higher states of consciousness. We turn next to the inner and outer mental being, an aspect of ourselves that rules, and is capable of guiding us through, the pitfalls of the subconscient; when enlightened, this aspect can utilize the subliminal and higher mental fields with great wisdom.

10
MENTAL BODY CONSCIOUSNESS

We want to know how to live well, and for this we must learn how to think well. To realise the primary importance of thought, we must know it as it is, as a living being....A little observation will enable us to realise that very often, for example, we receive thoughts which come to us from outside, although we have not been brought into contact with them either by speech or reading...a thought which is "in the air" as we say...thought which is a dynamism in the highest sense of the word, acts in its own realm as a formative power in order to build a body for itself. It acts like a magnet on iron filings. It attracts all the elements which are akin to its own character, aim and tendencies, and it vivifies these elements—which are the constituent cells of its own body, that I call fluidic...it animates them, moulds them, gives them the form which is best suited to its own nature.

-The Mother (Alfassa, 2003, pp. 88-90).

From this viewpoint, thoughts are living entities—especially those thoughts which have been given some power. Thoughts have consequences. The Mother asks us to consider:

If you reflect upon the incalculable number of thoughts which are emitted each day, you will see rising before your imagination a complex mobile, quivering and terrible scene in which these formations intercross and collide, battle, succumb and triumph in a vibratory movement which is so rapid that we can hardly picture it to ourselves. (Alfassa, 2003, p. 91).

The vibratory resonance field of mental consciousness focussed at the third level of the human energy field and interwoven throughout our being, the *mental biofield* reverberates with thought-forms. This bombardment of thoughts encodes a multidimensional resonance system that impacts each and every cell in the body right down to the genetic level.

The new science of epigenetics tell us how this gene-based, dynamic system of feedback loops either supports coherent healthy states of being or initiates grooves of negative coding that can ultimately lead to dis-ease. Sri Aurobindo pierces any lackadaisical perceptions with the reminder:

> Much more than half our thoughts and feelings are not our own in the sense that they take form out of ourselves...a large part comes to us from others or from the environment. (Sobel, 2007, p. 47).

The Mother elaborates:

> All the thoughts of worldly-minded people whose only aim is enjoyment and physical diversion, express craving. All the thoughts of intellectual creators or artists thirsting for esteem, fame and honor, express craving. All the thoughts of the ruling class and the officials hankering after more power and influence, express craving...we must learn to resist this daily pollution victoriously... If from place to place there occasionally flashes out a spark of pure and disinterested thought, of will to do well, of sincere seeking for truth.... (Alfassa, 2003, p. 92).

Sincere seeking that leads to a wisdom-centered advocacy for humanity is to be supported. Those who can sincerely seek for truth are, she says, "stars that one by one will come to illumine the night" (p. 92).

Aspiration, rejection, and surrender are the master keys to the psycho-transformative process that kindles these stars (Ghose, 1996): an aspiration that seeks connection with soul and spirit, a rejection that grows in discernment involving the inner being, and a surrender focused solely on Thy Will, as the Mother so poignantly reminds us. Sri Aurobindo says:

> You have only to remain quiet and firm in your following of the path and your will to go to the end. If you do that circumstances will in the end be obliged to shape themselves to your will, because it will be the Divine will in you. (Dalal, 2007, p. 29).

For our purposes here, *sadhana* is considered a process of active, conscious, working toward unveiling the psychic being or soul so it can provide guidance (Dalal, 2007). Applying the master keys underlying the evolutionary process supports psycho- transformation. Aspiration must be fixed and unfailing, we are told—it must have a strong, sustaining will supporting it. There must be a sincere willingness to surrender all parts of one's being, a constant and detailed awareness (to the degree possible) of truth as it is presented, and then conscious choice in all things, big and small. Rejection includes rejecting all that leads from the light, truth, and coherence: all falsehood. This rejection includes seeing beneath situations, seeing behind appearances and around appearances, and knowing when one is most vulnerable, either from within or from adverse forces acting from without (Pandit, 1992).

Armed with the master keys that serve as principles for action and as processes that unfold over time, the inner prompting to bow to soul guidance (more and more serenely and with surety) slowly informs the outer consciousness— this is the essence surrender, and of the healing process itself. The mental being's role is to provide an increasingly conscious process of harmonization, of ensuring that all (or as much as possible) of one's force is centered in the soul, and thereby, that the Beyond-ego nature is activating. Healing occurs when the notion of the deep inner wisdom of the Divine is accepted by the outer mind with sincerity, and is allowed its own wise, patient, yet persistent evolutionary path. This path of Divine wisdom is particular to the context of each person's karma and dharma, and especially, their *svabhava dharma* or law of the personal nature (Ghose,1996; Dalal, 2007).

Healing and utilization of the outer mental nature initiates a different kind of journey when viewed from within the context of these master keys. The keys help us understand the meta-process inherent in discovering wholeness—a process of purification and consecration (Dalal, 1999). Here, consideration is given to the outer and inner being, the subconscient and subliminal influence, and the development of the psychic being or soul consciousness. Extreme challenges associated with the process of health and healing from a physical viewpoint are discussed in the next chapter.

The thrust here is toward establishing a foundation for the mental body's role in the healing process based on four main Integral yoga mental-body derivations: physical-mind, emotional- vital-mind, thought-mind, and spiritual-mind. While there are many aspects to the mental body, and numerous derivations for discussion, when a fine and discerning view of Integral yoga is outlined, these four mind aspects provide a foundation for raising awareness pertinent to the inner and outer being, and the processes that nurture witness-consciousness.

Sri Aurobindo describes the physical-mind as

...that part of the mind which is concerned with the physical things only—it depends on the sense-mind, sees only objects, external actions, draws its ideas from the data given by external things, infers from them only and knows no other Truth.... (Sobel, 2007, p. 49).

The physical mind dominates the surface consciousness by utilizing the senses: what it can see, hear, smell, taste, and touch is real. It learns basic information, sets perceptions, and then utilizes these perceptions in rote or mechanical ways. Soon, entrenched cycles of behaviors and thought patterns monopolize the day.

In many ways this state of mind can serve; however, problems arise whenever a way-of-being becomes rote and blind to purpose and discernment. If, as the Mother warns, many of the guiding thoughts are from the environment and are mindlessly accepted as valid, then it is certainly not long before something happens in life to jar the mechanized system of responses. Moreover, the other aspects of the outer being or pressure from the inner being will tend to introduce corrective responses once an individual has gone too far off course.

Second, the emotional-vital-mind's role in Sri Aurobindo's teachings is to

> ...plan or dream or imagine what can be done. It makes formations for the future... [it] is a mind of dynamic will, action, desire—occupied with force and achievement and satisfaction and possession, enjoyment and suffering, giving and taking, growth, expansion, success and failure, good fortune and ill fortune.... (Sobel, 2007, p. 61).

Mental functions are here steeped in rajasic need, desire-based activity, and rationalizations that support needs and desires. The emotional-vital-mind caters to emotions, passions, desires, and ambition, and sets the longed-for outcomes into ideas that sustain mental forms. Sri Aurobindo warns that this, "the mind of desire and sensation, is the creator of the sense of evil...inherent in the form of pain and pleasure..." (p. 73). Emotional tyranny can enslave individuals and imprison right action, right thought, and free judgment when individuals are run by rajasic swings of attraction and repulsion. The aim of the emotional-vital-mind is to create a striving dissatisfaction and a general unrest.

The third major derivation of mind is the thought-mind.

Sri Aurobindo elaborates:

> The proper function of the thought-mind is to observe, understand, judge with a dispassionate delight in knowledge and open itself to messages and illuminations playing upon all that it observes and upon all that is yet hidden from it but must progressively be revealed, messages and illuminations that secretly flash down to us from... above our mentality whether they seem to descend through the intuitive mind or arise from the seeing heart. (Sobel, 2007, p. 81).

The function of this mind is to think, reason, perceive, consider, analyze, and allow for intuitive knowing. The thought-mind accesses ideas, places them within a cognitive framework, and when possible, includes vision and will. The thought-mind remains deeply connected to the senses and sensations; however, it keeps the witness stance awake. It works toward right understanding and responsible living, and is capable of utilizing higher order reasoning such as induction, deduction, inference, analogy, metaphor, and guided imagination along with disciplined judgment.

Intellect and faith can overlap so the 'thinker' does not become the 'thinking'—there is an ability to step back, disallowing the reign of the vital realms. However, the adverse forces and opposing suggestions from many realms can certainly interfere with the thought-mind. In order to uphold right thought and action, the courage to 'see' must be present along with a steadfast wisdom that allows inner-being promptings and higher- order insights. Here, the spiritual-mind aspect acts as guide since it is more permeable to spiritual and soul intimations.

Finally, the spiritual-mind has access to the outer-being and inner-being templates, but is focused on higher consciousness and a sacred view of Truth. Sri Aurobindo tells us that the spiritual-mind focuses on a "fire of purification, aspiration, devotion, true light of discernment..." (Sobel, 2007,p. 107).

The thought-mind holds the capacity for rational discerning states; however, as these two minds interlink, a space is held for inner discernment, illuminatory vision, and intuitive insight. With the spiritual-mind awake, there is a natural affinity for Truth. We are told that the ability to see through false appearance, disguise, and subterfuge is enhanced. The concealed Witness, or hidden guide, can then provide routes for deeper inner experiences. The power of inner vision is enhanced, sadhana is activated, and an inner silence separates itself from the rajasic and vital life-movements (or kinetic impulses), thereby permitting a sattwic calm that admits broader contextual perspectives.

Remaining true to yogic self-development and the power of experience, we now turn to representative examples of mental-body consciousness from my research (abridged from Lamb, 2010). The mental body in its complexity is master guide to the personality and to attitude, behavior, and action; if aligned to inner wisdom and connected to a healthy-enough egoic structure, the mental body can be mistakenly sabotaged by lower cunning aspects of the ego or false-self, or pirated by alternate forces set on destruction.

To focus on returning to mental-body consciousness, we consider selections from two clients who had strong mental fields used dually—sometimes to assist them in understanding and grasping what they needed to do to succeed, and other times to master-mind self-sabotage. Our first client, Ted, realized that he had used his 'own rebel thinking' to get him close to a complete breakdown. He was a highly functioning employee prior to the cascading, deteriorating, 'bottoming out' of acute addiction. Though naturally mentally astute, he became mentally unsettled, constantly overrode rational choices, and became extremely hyper, confused, and as he said, a complete 'scattered mess'. Here we see him gaining some tools, only to slip out of his body during healing sessions until he learns that healing occurs when he is in the body. The second client, Andy, listened this time in his treatment program and said he had become teachable. He grasped many ideas and brilliantly learned about his body energy and energy flows; nevertheless, we see how deeply pervasive intrusive energies combined with shame and guilt hold him, as they have potential to hold others to ransom.

We enter Ted's case at his second Integrative Energy Healing treatment, which the practitioner described as follows (Lamb, 2010, pp. 185-190).

> This past week Ted states he has been overwhelmed emotionally and mentally learning the tools he requires and needs to put in place when he leaves the treatment center tomorrow, in an effort to remain sober and drug free. He states that he wants to focus on his heart.
>
> He tends to project out of his body during treatments and states that he prefers to stay out of his body instead of communicating. However, he remains in his body for this treatment and could dialogue throughout. He is learning. Together we set the intention to balance his heart chakra and to call in the support that he requires at this time. During the treatment a technique to allow his energy field to relax, deepen, and open was used... I held the space and met him at the edge energetically and waited for him to allow me in. He then says "the heaviness in my heart is going." I ask him to think or express gratitude for his lessons, and he sighs and relaxes more and releases. He knows that he can make a conscious choice to replace what has left— his emotional energy field balanced and aligned. He chose to fill up consciously with the energy during this part of the treatment.

Note how Ted is aware that he consciously dissociates so not to connect with himself or others. This physical-mind- initiated rote defense mechanism is well established. However, to Ted's credit he allows his thought-mind to empower his awareness once the practitioner has established understanding and enough safety for him to experience embodiment while he is in an expanded healing mode. The practitioner continues:

Dialogue on how to discern and choose whose energy to take in, and when and where his lower-self is located, and how this part of him can test his intention was discussed. He points to the right side between the 2nd and 3rd chakras to identify the location of the lower-self. He is conscious of the tone of voice used and smooth talking style of this part of himself. He also points to his heart to identify the location of his higher-self.

Note: In the debriefing time for self-care, Ted speaks about taking energy from others when they are feeling burdened (his children) or fragile (substance-using friends). We discuss the awareness of bodily cues to sense when he is going off alignment or others are intruding on his space. Ted states that since he was a boy he has been aware of intrusive energies and does not know how to respond to them or what to do, but they do take him off his center. I discuss with him how to address these energies. After the treatment, Ted states he is feeling clarity, awareness, and control both emotionally and mentally, and is deeply calm, which is very different from how he felt when he arrived.

Ted states he reflected on our discussion last week about taking on another's energy and has become aware of how he has been doing this, especially with his children and friends. He witnessed himself 'feeding off' his daughter and vice versa, which made him realize that he was creating a problem instead of resolving an issue. He states this week he has made an effort to detach, to be present for himself, not giving himself away.

With very little theoretical information, Ted is capable of identifying how he uses his energy, and how he can misuse it or allow himself to be misused—he is aware that he himself is making the decision. The physical-mind aspect was well established as was his emotional-vital-mind's agreement to 'feed' off others at times, and at other times to let others 'feed' off him. But not until the treatment sessions had he activated the thought-mind aspect to reason through what he was doing to himself or to others. He chose to teach his daughter the biofield self-care strategies he was learning, thereby disrupting old patterns of behavior. The practitioner added:

> During one treatment Ted begins to see colors. While I am on his 3rd chakra he sees purple, he states that this color is coming from me and there is warmth to the color and he feels safe. The purple color continues until I come to his 5th chakra where it shifted to aqua. He states the aqua and purple colors represent strength to him. He states he is "in control of the colors" and is more conscious and aware while 'being' with the colors. After the treatment he states he had emotional and mental clarity.
>
> Ted goes home and returns for further sessions. His intention had been to maintain the calm he felt when he left the healing last week. It remained with him all week. He states it feels good to be home and he continues to feel strong and positive. States he has not used any substances and his resolve to remain sober is strong. He has been working daily and is feeling pain in his lower back. He and his daughter have been educating themselves reading material and grounding. He states he has been setting goals for himself at the start of the day

and this has helped him cope emotionally. When he has encountered an emotionally charged issue, he delays his response, and notices there is no charge to the issue when he does go back to resolve the conflict/issue. States he is sleeping well and is full of energy throughout the day, regardless of the back strain.

He receives a back treatment. The colors began immediately while I am on his legs. The first color he experiences is the sea green, like before, yet with more green. I ask Ted: "what do you need to know about the color?" He states "To integrate." This color stayed until I got to his 2nd and 4th chakras when the color turned to purple. Here the response is "pleasure", when I get to his arms, the affect shifts to "happiness". While going around his head, he states the purple coming in is intense and energy is flowing down his body and out of both of his feet. He says "I am an open vessel to receive." During the back treatment, he is silent for the duration of the treatment, except to state that the pain is draining out of his body on the left side and going into the earth. His pain started at 5/10 and shifted to a 2/10.

Ted's inner being opens and brings inner sight with it, he can 'see' colors and finds meaning-making words that assist him to utilize the experience throughout his mental-body. He is activating the thought-mind in ways that enhance the understanding of the emotional- vital-mind while continuing to keep the physical-mind safe, thereby he is able to change rote behaviors. He also enhances his skills at grounding such that he can release tension and pain himself, relieving himself of back strain and pain.

Self-care focuses on his increasing awareness of how he knows or understands energy. Ted states "my awareness of the energy is just on the edge of knowing." He is struggling to describe his relationship with colors. This leads to a discussion of how he can notice within his body when he is in alignment with the sky and earth. He also states that the energy coming in from the earth is "smooth" and the energy coming in from the sky is "vibrant and open." Additionally, I discuss the value of setting an intention at the beginning of the day and how this can set the tone for the day, as he says that he has more clarity at the beginning of the day and is drained at the end. We also discuss how he can use the earth connection to drain off the day's chaotic energy at the end of the day, and then to refill with vibrant energy.

He states that when he came into treatment on his first day he wrote in his journal, "My body is a vessel that is clogged. I need to let go and release." He states, "Today I did that." He continues to describe that he gets that insight now on a deeper level as he experiences the energy coming in from the sky and moving down his body, and conversely, up from the earth, through his feet and out the top his head. He is beginning to discern what is his energy field and what is another's. Ted also states he has "Crystal clear clarity that he is not going to use drugs again and that he is in control of choosing."

While many aspects of the inner and outer being and the body consciousness as a whole are activated, it is evident that Ted has gained a more discerning and structured plan of action to address numerous daily activities that could take him off his healing journey. He has empowered his thought-mind with concrete strategies that he is allowing himself to both understand and utilize. This process shows how impactful the thought-mind can be in relation to the emotional-vital-mind that has been steeped in satisfying the desires of the 'Reckless one' for some time. Later, the practitioner offered Ted a trauma- release treatment and he answered: "I am not strong enough to do the trauma release yet." The practitioner added:

> During discussion he says: "I am at one with myself. And I know this is what helped me. I know it has come from within me. You have guided me to help me remember." Ted said this with tears of gratitude. "I cannot drink or it will cloud my perspective. I get stronger daily."
>
> During the fifth healing session Ted is asked: What is working? What is not? He answers: "I am eating healthy and I am exercising. Everything is working. On the drive up country with my mother, thoughts of using came up, I always stop and use at this one place." He says that he was aware that this was his lower-self, and in being able to recognize this, his next thought was to wait for something better to come instead of being in reaction to his urge. He says he recognized it as a matter of choice. States he is open with his friends and family and coworkers and has received respect.
>
> What is helping? "Energy healings, yoga, breath work, mental awareness, the change in my energy, looking deeper into my soul, not having the same clouded vision, accepting imperfections, and my family is okay with my imperfections"; What is not working? "Nothing is coming up to complain about. Where I was is so different from where I am now. I am receiving daily rewards for where I am now"; Right now what do you need most to help you detox? "Being calm, being in charge of my day, being in control of my day"; Is there a new focus on life purpose? "The gains I am making with close family ties and close friends, my aura changes, others are responding positively to me, being respectful and honest. I have internal and external support and it is nice sharing life with people who support me";

Obstacles, what are they? "There are moments of being tested, which I realize goes with everything, therefore I need to be prepared and strong. I recognize I need a healthy body to have a healthy mind. I am not denying there is a potential—my house is in two names so 'he' does not have access to money to use"; Where do the obstacles arise? "It is my mind set…important not to overload myself by taking on more than I can handle"; Is there a struggle and strategies? "You get what you put in. Things are falling into place. Honesty to self, honesty as to why my intention is to be in recovery—stay drug and alcohol free and to go a lot farther with my energy healing—want to use the energy healing to open more doors and no traveling outside my body."

This discussion is followed with a series of healing protocols and a heart-balancing treatment and grounding. His head still tilts off to one side and in doing so he disconnects his alignment. I bring his awareness back to him again. He says, "Now my energy is more defined, it was sloppy at first."

His intention for the sixth healing is to ask for greater clarity about what he needs to know about himself. States he is feeling much stronger and is better able to do things in general. Physically he is still feeling muscle tension and continues to stretch daily. He is meditation and practicing his grounding and centering. Mentally he states he is not second-guessing himself. He says he is more disciplined, calmer and friendlier. He says his new life style is bringing him closer to his daughter. He has been teaching her grounding, centering and aligning to help her with her exams. He is using what he has learned from the energy healing sessions and interviews with Ruth in his life—it is the foundation and basis of his new lifestyle. States he is calm and doing things more methodically. States his desire to leap forward in great bounds has ceased, he can now remain calm by focusing on the earth's core. He realizes that practice and discipline will keep him grounded and calm. He knows his purpose is to be a responsible parent and he wants to remain in touch with energy healing and study what it is we do.

I did the sacred heart-based treatments and several bilateral balance treatments, with heart work to reaffirm this open receptive place. For the first time Ted got the importance of intention when he went into his heart space. He continues to see colors and to gain a sense of their meaning for him. He is able to feel his central channel from the earth to the sky. During the heart treatment he is surprised to learn that there were nooks and crannies in his heart that need to be cleaned out. He states that once the clearing happened he could have floated away, but he stayed and felt reborn and revitalized.

During self-care he notes that before he came into treatment, he was a 'lost soul' with no place or purpose, and he now knows his purpose is to be responsible and his place is to teach other addicts about Integrative Energy Healing. States: "I feel light" and he is ready to make more space. He did not realize there was more junk within and he will make time to clean out the junk from the spaces. "I needed to learn that." He says he is not in a hurry to clean out all the junk but he will know when he needs to. "I have never felt this way in my life, calm and content. I trust myself. I will know what I need to know, when I need to know it."

By his seventh healing Ted's intention is "to deepen my awareness of my physical body from the place of my heart." Life is going well. Ted has been asked to assist a family member with his son's substance abuse issues. His uncle says that when he looks at Ted's face, he knows he is doing well. Ted continues his integral meditations, his biofield exercises, and yoga and is working 12-hour days. Even during work Ted says he is able to relax himself both physically and mentally which is having a positive effect on his overall energy. Emotionally he feels well and can see the positive effect it is having on family and friends. States he saw his community drug counselor who gave him feedback, "Whatever it is you are doing, keep it up." He says that whenever he is feeling off or desiring a drink he thinks of the earth and lets the thought go and he feels okay. I knew my addiction was psychological but I did not know how to de-stress myself, now I do. My daughter is excited. What I am doing is coming back ten-fold."

When I am on his heart he says, "I know you cannot harm anyone from this place." Then he says, "I can travel around my body with my mind, this is the language of light, becoming more one with Self. Truth, my energy, and my honesty, are good things. This is old me revitalized with new tools. I am charged with life, my energy, and my family."

During self-care, Ted acknowledges his own wisdom, and is gaining confidence that all we worked on can be accessed by him at any time. His final comment below is why I do this work. Ted: "I was worried that this was the last healing session, but not anymore. I am at peace with who I am and where I am going. I am very happy about that."

Ted's return to heart-centeredness shows an activating spiritual-mind. This change brings a longing to connect more authentically, for example with his daughter, his other family members, and his colleagues. Ted activates his witness consciousness, regaining the wisdom to claim his limits while reconfiguring his old boundaries. He is inspired as he considers the 'new me', and has enough sattwic awareness to pace himself.

Ted says it all. He started out a 'scrambled mess' listening to the dictates of the well ensconced 'Reckless one's' sly suggestions that increased his addictive behaviors and increased his intake of coarse energies from the environment and from others who used. All this served to take him more and more off-course so that his job was lost, his house in jeopardy, and his family alienated. He was on the way to final destruction when pressure from within 'called' him back, and the healthy aspect of thought-mind and spiritual-mind that remained was able to access the needed assistance. That assistance included an acute addiction treatment center and a knowledgeable Integrative Energy Healing practitioner.

Ted's physical-mind and emotional-vital-mind routines and rote patterning gained a much needed redirection as the thought-mind and spiritual-mind interceded. New information and new understanding contributed to his success, accompanied by experiences that required new choices and renewed internal consent. His gain in witness-consciousness, if nurtured, can sustain ongoing supportive decision-making.

When trauma is initiated very early and when fathers and mothers fail their children and themselves, time is required for these sophisticated healing processes to be established. To reaffirm the ongoing biofield nature of trauma and the role of the mental-body, we take a glimpse into Andy's tenth healing as described by the practitioner (Lamb, 2010, pp. 191-193).

> The tenth healing intention, "To release guilt and shame, therefore achieve self-forgiveness and acceptance." Andy is early for his appointment. He talks about his eagerness and dedication to his healing. He worked every day this week painting. He is feeling really proud and good about that. He

also shares that he is now talking to his mother again, hasn't for the past year, and it feels great "to have mom's support is...like wholeness." But he also shares the enormous guilt and shame he feels about stealing and selling his mom's stuff. Andy recognizes the issue of boundaries...not wanting to say "Yes" to any family member, especially mom's requests, because of guilt. He wants to say it for the right reason. He expresses that he is feeling nervous/anxious and intimidated when he thought of going to a family dinner next week. "How could I let my family down the way I did with all the choices I made?" He feels horrible now about what he has done and some of his choices. And that is what he wants to work on for today.

During the treatment, there is a shape-shifting in his biofield right in front of my eyes. From the calmness/peacefulness he comes in with, to when he starts talking about the relationship with his mother. In his 1st chakra the energy becomes dense having formed into an actual cloud of compacted consciousness of guilt, making it vulnerable and thereby easy for the intrusive energy to attach itself there. 2nd chakra has bidirectional current, his 3rd chakra has an intrusive energy attached to it, the 4th chakra is rotating in a clockwise direction, his 5th chakra carries bidirectional current, the 6th chakra is congested/ cloudy and the 7th chakra is wide open. His energy field is lopsided, bulkier to his left side.

A treatment is given to promote and support healthy flow along his neural pathways and to improve grounding. Client appears to absorb the energy heart- fully. When my hands are under the 2nd chakra and left knee, the entity attached to the first chakra seems to fall off effortlessly as the vibrations increase. Then I do a heart balance to harmonize the vibrational qualities in the heart chakra. Slow to balance. Andy describes experiencing an inner state of alert stillness as he allows his energy field to fill. There followed a long silence...holding supporting and reinforcing the place of having a choice. I can sense integration, processing, and stillness. It was when the client entered 'an inner state of stillness' he detaches from the energy of guilt and the intrusive energy that is attached to his first chakra removes itself, effortlessly.

Client comments: "I feel really good about myself,confident about my own ability to make choices, saying Yes or No. I feel my self-worth. I am not scared of what might come up. I wish that the family dinner was tomorrow, rather than next week!"

Post-treatment assessment showed the 1st and 2nd chakra rotating clockwise, 3rd chakra still nesting the intrusive energy, 4th chakra rotating clockwise direction, 5th chakra has bidirectional current, 6th chakra rotating clockwise direction, and 7th chakra does not appear to have the same degree of openness. Self-care focuses on the practices of grounding and centering, and practicing awareness—he always has a choice. Also, he agrees to pay attention to the ways in which he expresses his truth, or not.

Andy went to the family dinner and later emailed his practitioner, "I have had a fall"—back to drugs. Two months later we heard he admitted himself to a recovery house.

The return of the mental body is fraught with challenges even though the clients here had a superficial cognitive grasp of the recovery process and could use the ideas they had learned to progress. With each client we get a glimpse of how the mind works to serve and to sabotage healing processes; however, with increased client understanding and willingness to change, combined with facilitated cocreative advanced biofield healing, much can be accomplished.

Early drug-use decisions impacted Andy's physical-mind; the grooves went deep and were reinforced by his environment and his friends' using activities. Even though the solace from drugs had long disappeared, the habitual, mechanical physical- mind sustained by the emotional-vital-mind served as a toxic recipe for disaster. Andy's previous stays in addiction treatment centres did not impact his thought-mind. He shared that in those days he felt he 'knew' better than his counselors, and "was in charge".

Today he has softened the old defenses and says he has become 'teachable'—a sign of thought-mind engagement. Concomitantly, his emotional-vital-mind is being governed by a wiser sense of self. Indeed, the spiritual-mind also engaged when Andy began to allow feelings of self-forgiveness and self- compassion. He is opening his heart. He can now acknowledge loneliness, grief, and guilt without collapsing. With each treatment, some progress was made as Andy allowed experiences that brought a deeper awareness of who he is and why he is here. He was able to examine what is working for him, and what is not working for him, and to be clearer with the differences. Even though he had a 'fall', he had enough awareness to put himself back in treatment within weeks rather than the usual years. He will face more of the war zone consciousness, but his time with more tools and a greater conscious awareness of Self.

What is required to support a growing sense of mental awareness from an Integral yoga perspective? The notion of healing as a conscious process places mind—that is, outer mind— in the forefront of awareness, because at this point the outer mind must be capable of choice and aware of the key processes, even if at a rudimentary level. Much sorrow, grief, fear, anger, and other strong disruptive emotions and desires tied tightly to beliefs that undermine wholeness can be—once there is a thought-mind awareness of a grander undercurrent that has meaning—unhooked from their emotional charge and quietly examined. That is, a separation from physical-mind rote behavior and the overriding of the emotional-vital-mind rajasic bring an awakening thought-mind that can differentiate reactions and select responses. Once the spiritual-mind is activated, added insights also support new behavior choices.

This differentiating and separating process births a witness consciousness that can step back and reflect—this is where the four aspects of the mental-being serve the healing process. Each has a role, and each can enhance or detract from any intention; once these aspects are understood, they nurture the witness. Individuals can now wisely consider themselves as many layered and many leveled beings. This awareness brings relief because when individuals step back somewhat, they tend to sense an inner core awareness, an aspect of themselves that remains steady, loving, and brilliantly supportive when they are able to access it.

Accessing this inner centre, psychic being, or soul brings a sense of peace and harmony—the attributes of healing. It is the activation of the psychic being, coming forth from behind the veil that often brings the ability to further the healing process by allowing individuals to identify with the uniqueness of their outer being while not allowing it to be the ruler of their destiny.

The ability to separate the mind from the emotions, and the emotions and mind from the physical body, is a valuable skill. Now individuals can grasp how each aspect of this outer- mental-being level impacts daily life—they can understand (or begin to understand) the battles and inconsistencies that have threatened their mental stability or health in general. This early understanding may be as far as some individuals can go depending upon the health of their ego structure. The Mother clearly states that one must be individualized—must know who one is—so one knows who is being surrendered to the Divine (Dalal, 1999).

Often called the process of self-realization, the individualization process is an aspect of Integral yoga and has many stages, as does mental-body consciousness in this context. Allowing the mental-body consciousness to access the psychic being and confirm its role and place is what establishes healing, again as a process, for the psychic being is the access point for all that holds the light (consciousness) for each person. Without the mental-body consciousness well aligned through all four aspects, the psychic being will remain buried deep within the innermost being, forced to work by subterfuge through coarse and deadened outer-being aspects and thereby having to utilize pain and suffering, dissatisfaction, and despair.

According to Sri Aurobindo, these inward subliminal, luminous, and concealed consciousnesses (e.g., the four mind- based perspectives) always influence us as does the psychic being (Dalal, 2007); however, becoming aware of their influence permits the individual to move inward, see more from an inward place, feel inwardly, and sense inwardly. While there are many challenges, drawbacks, and even risks to the old patterns of mental, emotional, and physical health in doing this, if the master keys are held tight as guiding principles, the journey brings greater mental awareness and a deep and abiding awareness of healing from a new, universalized, and harmonized perspective (Dalal, 2007).

Moving inward mentally also initiates an understanding of the role of the subconscient—the nether realm that holds automatic, unrefined, obscure, and submerged material capable of bringing havoc to all levels of health. The subconscient can certainly bring anguish and despair, depression, and many coping strategies that support repression (all to the detriment of immediate health). Yet, all these can also be turned and become the raw material and building force for an evolution of consciousness, a deeper awareness, an appreciation for the Divine plan and karmic process, and even an understanding of the severe testing that can accompany a willingness to heal (Sri Aurobindo, see Ghose, 1991).

Widening our frame of reference to include mental-body consciousness, let us turn again to the subpersonalities. Once established, the physical-mind brings a rudimentary subjective justification to consciousness and can limit aspects of the personality to constellations of subpersonalities when stress or challenging situations trigger the vulnerabilities that hold the subpersonality in place. The emotional-vital-mind works in tandem, solidifying and crystallizing the beliefs that hold the subpersonalities in

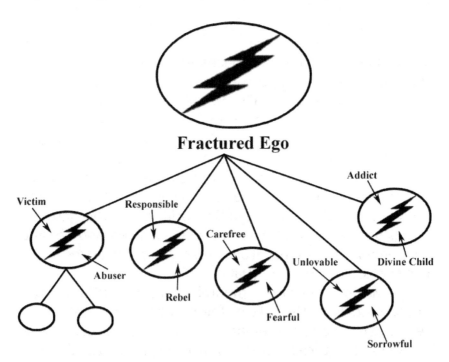

Subpersonalities.
Once there is enough emotional wounding to establish subpersonalities (split-off aspects of consciousness), the mental-body consciousness seeks to bring meaning to these aspects.

place. When the thought-mind activates, some degree of witness consciousness may be attained, but often not enough to resolve the actual subpersonality constellation.

In effect, mental awareness has been gained but the deeper healing process has not been engaged. Awareness is a valued first step, but nevertheless awareness alone does not stop the subpersonality from ruling behaviors. It is only when a deeper permission for healing, a sincere sense of safety, and an emotional softening of defenses has been attained that healing processes can engage. Once sufficiently engaged (often with facilitative external support and sustaining methods), the spiritual-mind consciousness brings the essential inner forces to the foreground—courage, resilience, and the will-to-change become possibilities. The journey to self-awareness can then take the next step. And with each step forward, with each gain in self-understanding and self-mastery, the egoic structure is given an opportunity to centralize, the personality to harmonize, and a new way of being to sustain.

Another factor to consider is the more consciously ascribed to persona or role aspects in our daily life, which tend to overtake the true inner personality if awareness slacks or rajasic business arises and seizes control. See the figure below.

Even with a healthy enough and centralized egoic structure, challenges occur as individuals attempt to live correctly, fulfilling role after role. When roles become fixated and overtake the natural harmonizing and balancing powers of the personality, we call this fixated role a persona or a mask. Once fixation occurs, it is relatively easy to lose touch with the centralizing egoic place of individuation and instead become the 'role'. For example, seeing oneself mainly—or even only—as a mother, father, son, daughter, grandmother, grandfather, professional, friend, or another title can become all consuming. It is even possible to get lost in the notion of an archetype such as healer, savior, rebel, victim, bully, soldier, president, prime minister, queen, king, and so on.

If more life force is spent in role fixation than is taken in, exhaustion occurs. From the emotional-vital-mind it can be viewed as discouragement, frustration, anxiety, or depression. From the physical-mind, the primal rajasic push to fulfill something that has become all consuming leads to low energy, fatigue, illness, and even chronic illness. The thought-mind at this point has succumbed to the role and is preoccupied with role-fulfillment at the cost of health and wellbeing. However, the shadow of this lifestyle brings boredom and rote mechanical life patterns that start to feel hollow and lacking in real meaning; the true value of the role has been lost when individuals 'become' the role. When this goes too far, the spiritual-mind becomes immersed in degrees of existential angst or actual despair, while at the same time it is in denial of the spiritual or sacred cosmic side to existence.

This is often the point at which a subtle or not-so-subtle push from the soul activates. If individuals permit themselves to seek a broader and deeper meaning to life—if

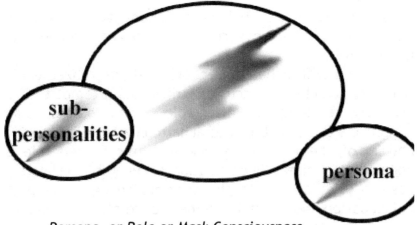

Persona, or Role or Mask Consciousness
The persona, often called the role or mask consciousness, can overwhelm as multiple roles in life compete with a balanced lifestyle.

they will allow the thought-mind to expand and reexamine life patterns—new understandings can arise. With its higher view and compassionate stance, spiritual-mind can assist individuals to place their roles into proper and respectful perspectives such that the true nature of the person can shine, and responsibilities can be fulfilled with a creativity and harmony that brings rather than drains life-force.

The aim of this yoga is to guide the formulation of a healthy enough outer mental-being such that there are increasing degrees of awareness of the subtle subpersonality linkages and pulls that drag on the centralized egoic structures. This awareness requires a witness or noticing understanding allowing individuals to access the inner-mental, subliminal, more powerful forces. These forces can enable the centralized egoic structures or disable the centralizing structures by empowering the more negative destructive subpersonalities or conglomerates of negative emotions to rule. One needs to activate the innermost soul wisdom utilizing the thought-mind perspective when daily challenges arise, and more forcefully, during times of initiation.

An empowered outer mental being with thought-mind awake can slow the destructive outpourings of the negative subpersonalities. The door is closed, the negative forces are disempowered, rejected, diffusing the enticing subterfuge of the subpersonality constellations and their nucleus of charged beliefs and values. The master keys, and methods and practices that sustain master key force, offer considerable influence and can initiate early intervention, especially with thoughts, emotions, and behaviors—once the decision has been made and the choice- points activated. A higher order idea can re-pattern low frequency sets that disarm integrity and lower the hierarchical placement of consciousness, thereby lowering the decision- making power, compromising decision-making, and bringing paths that lead to further destruction.

The thought-mind and spiritual-mind working in

conjunction have the power to impact or reset the mental-body consciousness to higher order frequency patterns that heal. This process, from a larger perspective, is a form of sadhana—a reaching for self-realization. In fact, it is a process designed to surpass the ordinary normal considerations pertinent to how we use our mental field and to how we see wholeness in general.

With regard to this point the Mother says: "...not a single person is normal, because to be normal is to be divine" (Alfassa, 1978, p. 292). This new evolutionary-based 'normal' places us in the centre of Integral yoga: lifetime after lifetime holding the master keys, hopefully with more assurance, awareness, trust, and humility, while maintaining an abiding faith in an absolute ground of Truth (Brahman).

As Sri Aurobindo states, there is an ancient promise that the Divine in each person will dissolve into the great Divine while maintaining a personality that can still function in Service—the psychic being will lead and Spirit will inform. In terms of the mind itself, Sri Aurobindo reminds us that "a still mightier Mind working in Life and upon it has not yet made sufficient way because the investigation of the laws of Mind is still in its groping infancy" (Ghose, 2007, p. 5).

In summary, the four aspects of the mental-body consciousness impacting both the inner and outer consciousness requires a constant conscious harmonization of the being at all levels and on all planes to the maximum possible. Hence, the healing process requires that challenges be accepted, faith upheld, and knowledge of the process reaffirmed time and time again while walking the soul-centered path of human becoming. Mastery of the key principles is ongoing, with a deep certitude that the soul will come forward and Spirit will guide. This unique harmonization must reach deep down into physical consciousness. As Sri Aurobindo explains the complex factors involved:

The first or superficial view which the observing mind takes on any object of knowledge is always an illusory view; all science, all true knowledge comes by going behind the superficies and discovering the inner truth and the hidden law. It is not that the thing itself is illusory, but that it is not what it superficially appears to be; nor is it that the operations and functionings we observe on the surface do not take place, but that we cannot find their real motive-power, process, relations by the simple study of them as they offer themselves to the observing senses. In the realm of physical science this is obvious enough and universally admitted. The earth is not flat but round, not still but constant to a double motion; the sun moves but not round the earth; bodies that seem to us luminous are in themselves, non-luminous; things that are part of our daily experience, color, sound, light, air are quite other in their reality than what they pretend to be. Our senses give us false views of distance, size, shape, relation. Objects which seem to them self-existent forms are aggregates and constituted by subtler constituents which our ordinary faculties are unable to detect. These material constituents again are merely formulations of a Force which we cannot describe as material and of which the senses have no evidence. Yet the mind and the senses can live quite satisfied and convinced in this world of illusion and accept them as the practical truth—for to a certain extent they are the practical truth and sufficient for initial, ordinary and limited activity... there are possibilities of a wider life, a more mastering action, a greater practicality which can only be achieved by going behind these surfaces and utilizing a truer knowledge of objects and forces. (Ghose, 2007, pp. 10-11).

This unique 'going behind' must reach deep down into physical consciousness. With this reassuring and rather intriguing encouragement to look deeper and behind the surface, we turn next to the physical-body consciousness and then subtle physical-body consciousness.

11
PHYSICAL-BODY CONSCIOUSNESS

The body is not mere unconscious Matter: it is a structure of a secretly conscious Energy that has taken form in it. Itself occultly conscious, it is, at the same time, the vehicle of expression of an overt consciousness that has emerged and is self-aware in our physical energy- substance. The body's functionings are a necessary machinery or instrumentation for the movements of this mental inhabitant; it is only by setting the corporeal instrument in motion that the conscious Being emerges, evolving in it can transmit its mind formations, will formations and turn them into a physical manifestation of itself in Matter.
-Sri Aurobindo (Dalal, 2001, p. 67).

Understanding this 'secretly conscious Energy' requires building a sophisticated awareness and a witness consciousness— a consciousness well worth developing. As we have seen, Sri Aurobindo and the Mother discuss a wide range of consciousness states including inconscient, subconscient, physical body- consciousness, vital consciousness, mental (lower) conscious, as well as the spiritual dimensions of higher mind, illumined mind, intuitive mind, overmind, supermental consciousness, and subliminal and psychic or soul consciousness (Ghose, 1996, 2000c; Alfassa, 2005). All states have different degrees of evolutionary potential and vibrational intensity, and of course, within each state there are substates. In this chapter we discuss physical health, illness, and healing by focusing on the lower mechanical-physical, emotional-vital-physical, mental-physical, and spiritual-physical consciousness.

Physical body-consciousness, or mechanical-physical consciousness is the most material, matter-like consciousness and is closely associated with earth-consciousness. It is steeped in centuries of habit, highly resistant to change, and opposed to transformation. This body-consciousness influences cellular consciousness.

While cells steeped in this resistant tamas are highly sensitive to emotional and mental suggestions, they also have an intensity for life, a desire to function well, an aspiration, and a will that wants to establish equilibrium. Left on their own without interference from the vital, the mental, or the environment, and left free from diagnostic categories already crystallized on the planet, cells will choose balance, harmony, and maximal health within the individual's karmic potential. Nevertheless, how individuals respond to life events dramatically affects the cells, leaving them vulnerable to dysfunction (Satprem, see Enginger, 1993).

As we have seen, emotional-vital consciousness grounded in desire (i.e., excess, passion-based consciousness rushing toward need-satisfaction) is easily caught in a cycle of anxiety, fear, obsession, compulsion, and depression. This consciousness is also led astray by suggestions carried by intrusive or hostile forces, whether from within or without (Pandit, 1994, 1999). Mental consciousness with its ideas, notions, concepts, principles, precepts, and dogmas impacts daily life. Much is unconsciously absorbed from the environment, home, school, family, workplace, the media, and becomes habit.

Together the vital and mental have tremendous influence on our lives, particularly the well-being of the physical body. When a false belief is powered by the emotional-vital, the Mother says the slave-oriented body-consciousness succumbs— the cells listen, obey, and their natural wisdom is forced aside. In fact, it is this habit of acquiescence to set belief structures that leads Sri Aurobindo (Ghose, 1996) to say that he prefers to work directly with symptoms rather than diagnoses, thereby bypassing crystallized thought-forms carried by the power of the diagnostic label itself. The challenge is to find ways of utilizing the diagnosis in treatment without having clients placed in a freeze-fear state through over-focus on the label.

According to the Mother (Alfassa, 1998), illness is created by the body-consciousness getting caught in a wrong attitude. For someone to be vulnerable to an illness and have the illness establish itself, the Mother says there must be a dislocation internally or externally. Internal vulnerability can be caused by fatigue, fear, shock, or depression.

Specifically, fear can become a huge determining factor that works to undermine the individual either consciously or unconsciously. If fear enters the subconscient, it goes underground and attacks from many angles. If it is conscious, the mind combined with the vital may choose to ruminate, constantly reworking the worst possibilities. This ruminating process may or may not be adversely aided by healthcare professionals, family or friends, and media or literature. If exacerbated, this state opens the door to greater disequilibrium manifesting as further pathology or an accident.

The original break in equilibrium can occur at the cellular, vital, mental, or subtle levels, consciously noted or not. However, once a disease process is fully installed in the subconscient's obstinate memory, even if it is apparently cured, it can easily return—until the root cause is addressed. When pathology confines itself mainly to the body-consciousness, the Mother terms the dysfunction either organic or functional. Organic dysfunction involves the organs directly while functional refers to the more serious systemic or multisystem disease pathology (Alfassa, 1998). Here, we use four specific lenses to examine physical-body consciousness: mechanical or material- physical, emotional-vital-physical, mental-physical, and spiritual-physical.

At the material-physical level, body consciousness is closely bound to the subconscient and to automatic physiological functions, closely tied to the primal brain's safety and survival- seeking responses. These responses overlie the physiological responses designed to protect, creating grooves leading to passivity.

Sri Aurobindo outlines the issue of physical-consciousness defects:

> There are many but mainly obscurity, inertia, Tamas, a passive acceptance of the play of wrong forces, inability to change, attachment to habits, lack of plasticity, forgetfulness, losing experiences or realizations gained, unwillingness to accept the light or to follow it, incapacity (through tamas or through attachment or through passive reaction to accustomed forces) to do what it admits to be the Right and the Best. (Ghose, 2000b, p. 1434).

The material-physical is closely aligned to the physical earth-nature, which is slow and inert so as to maintain a much needed planetary stability. Still, inertia plagued by chaos impacts both the earth-nature and individuals. The combination of tamas and chaos, especially when it occurs over and over, creates grooves in the material-physical and can pass through a family or heritage line into character and body traits—especially if the emotional-vital has been impacted, as with trauma factors. On the other hand, strong and positive life-affirming traits can be transmitted as well. This mix includes the issues of Nature and Nurture, and of course, ideas related to karma and reincarnation in the Vedic sense, discussed in Part Three.

Connected directly to the physiology of the nervous system, the emotional-vital-physical is a place that can hold joy and peacefulness but is more often clouded by obscure desires. Sri Aurobindo tells us that this is the most "animal part of the human being" (Ghose, 1995, p. 1423) but it is not to be despised. He says, "it is part of the intended manifestation" (p. 1423) and counsels the following.

> One has to come in contact with it so as to know what is there and transform it. Most sadhaks [seekers] of the old type are satisfied with rising into the spiritual or psychic realms and leave this part to itself—but by that it remains unchanged, even if mostly quiescent, and no complete transformation is possible. You have only to remain quiet and undisturbed and let the higher Force work to change this obscure physical nature (p. 1423).

It may be this very physical body consciousness, in its emotional-vital aspect couched in reticence, that brings the much-spoken-of 'dark night of the soul'. According to Sri Aurobindo:

> There is a certain...critical stage through which almost everyone has to pass and which usually lasts for an uncomfortably long time but which need not be at all conclusive or definitive. Usually if one persists, it is the period of darkest night before the dawn which comes to every or almost every spiritual aspirant. It is due to a plunge one has to take in to the sheer physical consciousness unsupported by the true mental light or by any vital joy in life, for these usually withdraw behind the veil, though they are not as they seem to be, permanently lost. It is a period when doubt, denial, dryness, greyness, and all kinds of kindred things come up with a great force and often reign completely for a time. It is after this stage has been successfully crossed that the true light begins to come, the light which is not of the mind but of the spirit. (Ghose, 1995, pp. 1426).

Regarding the mental-physical level, Sri Aurobindo cautions that mental awareness is not enough:

> Hitherto your soul has expressed itself through the mind and its ideals and admiration or through the

vital and its higher joys and aspirations; but that is not sufficient to conquer the physical difficulty and enlighten and transform Matter. It is your soul in itself, your psychic being that must come in front, awaken entirely and make the fundamental change. (Ghose, 1995, p. 1424).

Here, the challenging spiritual-physical aspect intersects with the overall physical-body consciousness. Integral yoga's notion, as presented here, of Consciousness, Force, Energy, Light, and Information resonates from the macro Absolute while taking us into the cellular and beyond to the micro-levels of the material-physical—in other words, to the level that the new epigenetic science addresses. The ancient yogas take us to that same level with their emphasis on hope and faith, peace and deep calm, and a heightened inspiration and sacred devotion. These modes and moods of being impact the whole person— the outer being and the inner being. This multidimensional to deep cellular, even genetic, imprinting comes with both beneficent and maleficent outcomes depending on what is present in the moment, what resilience and skills we have to meet each challenge, and what patterns of response are well established due to past history, as well as many other factors still in the realm of mystery.

From this view, dimensions of becoming always call us back to the integral nature of the human condition. Not only does the soul journey get disrupted, but actual physical health gets disrupted when life experience takes us away from the state of 'Know Thyself'—that is, the higher self or soul connection.

Let's examine the third focus, mental-physical, in detail. Many aspects of the mental-physical are automatic and completely helpful in steering our physiology correctly and sustaining a maximum state of wellbeing. The amazing miracle of our physical-body consciousness closely relies on the material- physical, emotional-vital-physical, and mental-physical to remain in dynamic equilibrium (Ghose,

1996, 2000b). When they are in a harmonious state, the best possible physical health is maintained; however, once disruption occurs in any of these three aspects, the body physiology responds. In terms of the mental-physical, Sri Aurobindo says it is an obscure mentality or mind that reaches to the very molecules, a mind that runs on habitual encoded pathways (Ghose, 2000b). Healthy habitual pathways serve us well, but disruption is capable of creating new pathways—for example, stress pathways. One must work to get rid of the doubts, anxiety, and inertia of the "physical mind, the defective energies of the vital physical (nerves) and bring instead the true consciousness..." (Ghose, 2000b, p. 1432).

Given this wise counsel, let's turn now to findings from new science—what the yogis experienced, and what Sri Aurobindo so carefully teaches, is becoming the language of modern science. We hear now that the physical is the home of programmed beliefs that act as friend or foe. If we are awash with fear-activated stress hormones, we cycle from flight to fight to freeze—a process that sets hormonal pathways into action (Dispenzia, 2007; Doige, 2007; Lipton & Bhaerman, 2010). From our view these pathways create grooves in the emotional- vital physical and the material-physical consciousness, and those grooves code for the stress response. If stresses are repeated, this process becomes hypersensitive and soon even minor irritants bring a full cascade of stress-related hormones. The nervous system is out of balance.

Of note, and often of grave concern, is the long established finding that experiences from birth to six years shape our response or reaction-program. Indeed, approximately 5% of our behavior is within conscious awareness via the outer being's nature; the remaining 95% is in the subconscient, invisible to us (Lipton & Bhaerman, 2010). As discussed above, the subconscient has direct access to all aspects of the outer being—what is more, the subconscient remembers everything that has happened to us, (Ghose, 2000b). This remembering is also held in the physical body at each level (the material-physical, emotional-vital- physical, and mental-physical). These three aspects amalgamate in their complexity, with direct links to the limbic and amygdala system of the brain: When we go on autopilot, for better or worse, we are in direct contact with these systems. Hence, a surprising 95% of our cognitive activity emanates from the subconscient (Lipton & Bhaerman, 2010). The subconscient has an awesome capacity to process information at 40 million nerve impulses a second, while the self-conscious, awakened, outer mental has the capacity to process only 40 nerve impulses a second. The inner being, from a subconscient perspective, is as powerful as the centuries old yogic science claims.

Interestingly, new science places a renewed focus on ancient teachings (Lipton & Bhaerman, 2010). Prerecorded subconscient programs hold a firm grip on individuals—Sri Aurobindo's yoga explains why 'talk therapy' can be quite useless and even why reasoning with someone is often equally useless. As we saw with the research clients drugging, of any type, is at best palliative (Lamb, 2010). Claiming the right to remember, to feel, and to speak is imperative. Honoring the story is a necessary route to re-storying, once a higher vibrational witness-consciousness can override and recode the well-worn physical body consciousness's behavioral pathways.

New science posits that the mind (or, from our view a complex system of minds) controls health, and that the mind controls gene function. Perception rules a large percentage of our behavior. Scientific research shows that the nervous system (directly linked to the emotional-vital-physical outer being) and the cells (actual material-physical consciousness) do not question information received either from the mental-physical or from the other aspects of being. Instead, they respond to life- affirming or life-destroying perceptions (Lipton & Bhaerman, 2010). Moreover, research shows that up to 70% of thought has negative overtones.

As perceptions, these thoughts reach into every cell, and when they reach the cell, our epigenetic scientists tell us they have access to the genes and a genetic selection for proteins that encode genes. The instantaneous follow-up action impacts the nervous system, immune system, and endocrine system (Lipton & Bhaerman, 2010).

Once steeped in a newfound understanding, positive beliefs can integrate throughout the outer being and honorably connect to the inner being's wisdom, bringing a relearning of perceptions, a renewal of meaning, and a soul-centered meaning-making (The Mother, see Alfassa, 1998). If there is an integral Truth to the healing process, the interlinkages reach right to the DNA-RNA transduction levels and release a new and helpful cascade of neurotransmitters and hormones. If this new process can be sustained, over time new patterns are recognized, new grooves for behavior set, and a new emerging paradigm of behaviors embraced. Sri Aurobindo reassures us:

> Transformation implies facing the difficulties and changing or overcoming what arises in each part of the being so that that part may respond to what is higher, but the full change of the whole can only come by the ascent to the Above and the descent from Above. (Ghose, 2000b, p. 1433).

Otherwise, we stay stuck in the physical consciousness in a state of "fundamental passivity in which one is and does what the forces of the physical plane make us do." (p. 1433).

Dis-ease leads to suffering whether it is physical, emotional, mental, or spiritual, and the Mother suggests removing the psychological root of the suffering (Alfassa, 1998). One of two types of suffering outlined by Sri Aurobindo, egoic suffering occurs when the individual feels violated by symptoms related to outer-being disequilibrium; the other, centered in the heart, is suffering associated with an inner-being divine compassion that feels the struggles of the world. If the suffering is the first type, egoic due to outer-being disequilibrium, the Mother suggests seeking and removing the wrong attitude by carefully examining conscious and subconscient tendencies related to outer aspects of the physical, vital, and mental behavior patterns and beliefs. When it is the second, suffering related to inner-being related compassion, she recommends bringing in the yogic process, using intuition and silence, freeing oneself from the outer mixed vital desires and mental superficial egoic notions, and deepening the soul connection, all of which leads to a broader understanding of the Divine in action (Sri Aurobindo & The Mother, see Ghose & Alfassa, 2006).

Inner Force Alignment

Primary: Initial response * Place force of consciousness on physical discomfort and increase cellular receptivity to higher vibrations of consciousness	* Reduce receptivity to the dissonant force(s)
Secondary: Ongoing response * Examine self for hidden corners of being that might be granting permission to false consciousness (dis-ease)	* Inquire at deeper levels of being, addressing dharma and karma by seeking meaning and opportunities for self-mastery

The Mother also notes a positive side to suffering in that it can bring a person out of inertia, re-awakening a new urge to heal by forcing the person to address disharmony (Alfassa, 1998). Once one is fully aligned with the decision to heal, the Mother outlines two methods to bring about a cure and specifies a four- step response to address adverse forces (Ghose & Alfassa, 2006). These methods are self-care strategies, not meant to take the place of additional health care. The first method of cure is to place the force of consciousness and sense of truth on the physical discomfort and increase cellular receptivity. Second, reduce receptivity to the inner affinity or correspondence that left the body open to disease, karmic or otherwise.

If the disease remains, she believes there is a deeper inner permission being granted or some affinity perhaps held in the inconscience or subconscient; or, she says, there are times when a disease is necessary for a person's development. Even so, to truly cure a resistant disease such that it does not return, a radical change of character is necessary. One must, she admonishes, hunt for hidden and darkened corners of the self harbouring the false consciousness that grants permission for disequilibrium— even to the point of sincerely addressing ideas of karma and dharma (Ghose & Alfassa, 2006).

Here is a story from my own life that reflects some of these steps. A 100-year-old family member living in a care- support facility has always been highly sensitive to energy fields and to her body-consciousness. The facility was on quarantine due to the Roto virus: as long as no one on your floor had the virus, family members could come in and individuals could go on outings. We went weekly to take our family member on outings that she really enjoyed. Planning ahead for the possible attack of the virus, she asked us to take her to a store to purchase a large clove of garlic, as she has always believed that garlic is a great immune booster and for years had used it in that way. In her opinion, she was armed.

On our return the following week we noted the garlic was gone. When we asked her what had happened, here is what she said: "I took the full clove of garlic when I noticed my throat tickling a bit; then I stayed away from others for a few days. At that time I noticed a dark cloud of viruses coming into my room— I demanded it leave immediately". She was alert to the subtle energy cloud made by the virus as it entered her room. She fiercely demanded the virus leave and took her trusted remedy. She and the whole floor of ten rooms were left free of the virus, which was highly debilitating to the point of taking lives. Care staff later told us that she lived on the only floor in the facility that did not experience the virus.

She may have been the only one on that floor who was not immunized, and certainly among the few in the building; however, the whole floor escaped the virus. Consciousness had to be directed immediately, and with diligence, and the Force of peace, stillness, and harmony combined with an inner refusal. She innately knew this process, and never missed an outing!

Turning now to our clients and practitioners who explored this unique focus on healing in my research, Luke and Jasper present some classic signs of physical-body consciousness holding-patterns. With a childhood of remembered alcohol- induced rage from his father and alcohol-induced shaming from his mother, Luke had almost succumbed to a heart attack due to his escalating cocaine use—this brought him into treatment. In childhood he could never be sure he was safe, or even okay. This warm hearted and fully employed man choosing not to repeat his parents' behavior towards others had repressed his own feelings of rage and shame, anger and frustration. His material-physical body and his emotional-vital-physical consciousness adapted: his body became hard and sore, causing him chronic back and neck pain and overall body pain. Alcohol and drugs maintained the wounding, providing solace for a time.

Let's visit Luke's healing experience as the practitioner described it (abridged from Lamb, 2010, pp. 169-176).

My general first impression of Luke is that he has soft lovely energy. This impression grew over the session as I sensed him coming into himself. On scanning his biofield he has low energy over his body. It feels from my hand scan and then my sense about him that most of his energy is above his head with very little in his body. There is a deeper disconnect at his pelvis and down his legs. I sense he is in a fragile state. As he discusses his intake assessment with me I note his desire to get well and to find strength in doing what it takes. His physical body is a little hunched, it seems compressed to me. He is a fairly large and is a strong looking young man.

The session starts with me asking him to allow thoughts to float away while he focuses on taking some breaths into his body, including his legs. After a few purposeful breaths, I sense he is a bit more present, I suggest he allow his body to breathe itself and remind him that his body is wise and knows what to do. I suggest he let gravity take over and let the table support him. As he did this I start clearing his field. I sense him come into his body a little deeper. While holding his 2nd and 4th chakra I am unable to connect with his field and his field does not respond by taking up any energy. I move to hold the back of his heart and his high heart area and sense after a time, some flow between these points. I then move to his head and offer his field a release technique. Initially I sense no flow moving down past his neck. Halfway through this technique his dural membranes start releasing very obviously. I can feel more space opening up and more energy flowing allowing the releasing to naturally pattern down his spine. This works very well in opening up the flow of energy down to his coccyx, although the flow is much weaker below the waist. Moving into a full body connection technique, in order to further open up the flow of energy in his field, I sense at each step a slow gradual balancing between the points being held. At his heart level 4th chakra, his field is not ready to open up. Flow is decreased here. While holding his heart area I ask him what he is noticing. He says that "every place you put your hands is where I have been sore." When asked how they were now he says "they feel much better." When I was holding the back of his heart and his high heart, he could "feel a flow of energy between the points." This seems to make him happy, almost like he is making progress.

By the end of the treatment there is still a lot of dense heavy energy being held in his body, but now there is energy flow around him. I sense him more in his body and also fairly calm and relaxed. I believe it is not so easy for him to be in his body and relaxed. He agrees that he feels calm and relaxed. He likes the idea of giving himself over to gravity. This helps him stop his mind chatter a bit and to be aware of his body. Grounding into the earth is discussed but Luke did not get a sense of this. For now just a sense of being in his body is a very good start.

By the third treatment Luke's intention is to continue grounding and being present. The practitioner commented:

His biofield at the back is quite tight and he has chronic neck and shoulder pain. A large area around the heart has a very dense area about 2 feet long sticking out the back. I then spend about 10 to 15 minutes working on opening up his back from top to bottom holding the back of his heart chakra and then connecting it to his 2nd chakra, shoulders and the front of his heart chakra. I sense more movement in his back than I have at any other time in the last two sessions. His heart area feels like my hand is sinking right into it. The 2nd is similar but not as much. I feel a flow of energy moving up and down his back and moving around in the heart chakra. Luke says, "I can feel the pain moving around and coming and going." I encourage him to just let it do that, and breath it out and release. He did that for the remainder of the treatment. Self-care includes quiet times in a quiet place and exercise. Breathing exercises with grounding, centering and aligning and central channel breathing as well. Suggest he set intentions for each day when he wakes in the mornings.

During the fourth healing, Luke told the practitioner about a self-abuse habit of his that was secret. She listened and encouraged him to discuss it with his counselor. In her words:

Luke is continuing to gain perspective. He says, "I am creating a light." He has mentioned before that he is noticing, "My friends are not really my friends." These people are people that were in his life when he was 'using'. To all of the above I respond with encouraging words and with the intention to mostly listen. He appears to be doing quite well in his recovery. He mentioned he has had some using dreams but he does not feel the need to take drugs again. He tells me he has been practicing the breathing techniques, grounding and centering. He says, "It is helping with my concentration." It seems to me that Luke is becoming more present in his body more of the time. In this place of 'presence' there are issues of his that are surfacing. It feel at this session that Luke is more trusting of me and therefore willing to tell me about the habit as discussed above.

By his fifth healing treatment his biofield is opening, Luke has an insight. He realizes that he does not honor his own truth. He finds this amazing. He is noticing at a more meaningful level his responses to people and situations in his life when he does not acknowledge or say his truth. He is happy that he is realizing this and shocked at the same time. Throughout the rest of the conversation he would go between this state of amazement and back into frustration and anger when he gets insights related to honoring, or not, his truth in daily life. He is seeing what he is doing in all areas of his life. Energetically this is a big opening. In his words he has "more belief in how I feel." I certainly encourage him here saying he is on track and is doing very well with the practice.

During the whole Integrative treatment it feels like his field is ready to release tension and come into balance. It seems that the yoga session he just attended maybe set his field up for the releasing and balancing in our session. It is like the yoga had freed up blocks of holding but they stayed in his field. I sense while holding behind his heart area that his central channel is stronger than I have ever felt it. There is some restriction in his neck so I then do a dural release. There is an almost immediate opening in his neck, head and down his spine. After some smoothing out of his field I grounded him and then guided him through a meditation: at closure his field is full and light all over. He is aligned and his central channel charged.

After his seventh healing treatment Luke seems to be doing very well since the beginning of our sessions together. He is more in touch with how he feels and his boundaries. He seems to be aware of how other people's energy affects him and he has learned some self- regulation techniques to help keep present and centered when challenged. He is aware that he will have good days and bad days—like the rest of us—and that he really is doing well in his recovery. He is slowly taking time to clean his living space. As he talks about this it seems to correlate to his own deepening and clearing process. A real step forward, his mother an alcoholic who had been very abusive to him moved out about a week ago.

Luke later contacts me asking if he could continue with another practitioner as our commitment was complete. I agree that he can if there is a cancellation but no space became available (Lamb, 2010, pp. 169-176).

Luke learned that as a capable adult he can now learn new ways of being. As he began to trust the practitioner, he came into his body at the material-physical and emotional-vital- physical levels. He released painful cellular holding and thereby softened his body tissues. He allowed himself to feel and activated a noticing that requires not only mental-physical skills but also good emotional-vital skills and mental being awareness. He started to uncover old emotions and gained insights into his behaviors. He also felt free enough to share his secret self-harm behavior with the practitioner; this self-harm process may have developed to deal with the overflow of self-shame, rage, and frustration that even his escalating drug use did not contain. He agreed to discuss this with his counsellor—a very good start, as the secret was no longer hidden from his or his practitioner's view.

By the final session Luke had asked his mother to leave his apartment and was no longer living with her or the shaming statements she made to him or his friends when they visited. He was aware of the many nuances that go with his friendships and seemed capable of using more thought-mind abilities to name what leads to further gains for his life versus distractions, even destruction. Last we heard Luke was clean, looked well and healthy, and had accepted a position in another town.

As a child, Jasper lived with constant physical, emotional, and sexual abuse; at the time of the research he is a young man suffering from migraine headaches and Fibromyalgia. In treatment for the first time and newly out of the hospital after a suicide attempt (his third), Jasper is skeptical but willing to explore this healing approach. Let's hear from his practitioner (Lamb, 2010, pp. 172-176).

Jasper's first healing intention: To experience an energy healing treatment and see if it can help release muscle pain from Fibromyalgia. As I assess Jasper's biofield 'high strung' comes to mind; emotional field thin, surface, little depth; mental field—quick, chaotic, and buzzing. The edge of his field is sensed off body almost 1 meter, thin, quick, with a substantial edge about 30 cm off body; the top of his field greater than the bottom it has an inward imploded feel to it. There is an energy 'push' off the right shoulder and right side of neck, and down the midline of his body, from throat to groin; note heavy energy sitting slightly off body between left knee and left ankle. Sense energy releasing ('leaking') from Jasper's ankles, knees, hips, shoulders, elbows and wrists and sense energy movements on surface of substantial energy field edge, as scan passed over energy changed pattern, direction, and flow.

Sitting in chairs, I introduce Jasper to grounding and invite him to practice through visual/somatic imagery—feeling the pull of gravity. He reports being able to feel and sense himself grounding. Jasper reports he is able to soften in his heart area and center his awareness within a feeling of expansion, and he can connect upward through his crown.

An alignment treatment was used to smooth field, facilitate long line energy flow and assist removal of heavier energies to ground. Focus on surface of substantial edge, concentrate on sense of connection with field as energy is 'difficult' to engage or grasp with etheric fingers; once connected energy moves easily to ground. Star treatment to balance and integrate field which is slow to connect. Jasper appears calm and is breathing slowly. Sweep field from head to toe three times focusing on facilitating energy flow and grounded Jasper at feet, invite him to bring awareness to his feet. Jasper reports being able to sense flow of energy as a "current running from head to toes." Following there are still areas of heavy energy, the 'push' around right shoulder and right neck dissipated and there is a flow to the field. Some heavy energy remains off body over core and weakly pushing out from left shin. Self-care: Move back to sitting in chairs, debrief treatment. We practice grounding, centering and aligning again. Jasper finds the experience of grounding and centering to have tangible benefits...his blood circulation improves noticeably and he reports feeling more present in his body which also includes feeling pain in his wrists that he said was there but easily ignored at the start of the session. Jasper, "I do feel current flow down, my head feels lighter...I feel a lot calmer. I definitely feel less tension and pain. It's much easier to breathe. Somehow it helps me breathe out longer. My blood circulation is a lot better. My hands and feet are warm. This is not usual. I have trouble with my circulation and my hands and feet are usually cold."

Second healing, intention: To relieve pain in areas where he stores his stress. Jasper comments that his awareness of sensations within his body is improving. He notes that it is easier to ground, center and align in the room with me than when he practices by himself. The edge of the biofield is off body almost one meter on right side, close to body on left swirling, moving quickly, electric, difficult to define substantial edge; several areas of heavy, dense energy noted: over left shoulder; pushing out from right side of neck; over right hip; right knee and left knee. Heavy, less dense energy noted over both elbows and left wrist. Overall, his energy field is active with swirling clouds flowing to the ground chaotically. Etheric Alignment to integrate and clear field with focused 'stops' with intention to facilitate flow/release of energy. Noted 'pushing' out from right side of neck. Overall field more stable flow – substantial edge sensed ~30-45 cm off body. Areas of dense, heavy energy diminish around left shoulder and right neck dissipates; note a spiral flow to the field to ground. Jasper says that the pain in his right shoulder area is "a lot less" as is the headache that he began to notice at the beginning of the treatment. He remarks, "You don't know how wonderful it is to have warm feet. I will continue to practice."

Self-care: Jasper finds the experience of grounding and centering to have tangible benefits... his blood circulation improves noticeably and he reports feeling more present in his body. He will continue to work on his grounding, lying down and sitting, focusing on a sense of gravity on the body and noticing the sensations and effects of that practice. He will practice grounding, centering and aligning with deep belly breaths while lying down, sitting in chair, walking, and when in conversation with others. Notice what happens inside and how he feels at the time.

Comment: My impression is that he is focusing on the impact of the energy treatment and grounding, centering and aligning on the physical aspect of his being. He describes his usual response is to 'numb out' the pain, particularly with the pain he experiences in and around his head. Jasper's awareness of his body is now quite good, he appears sensitive to energy flow and, with minimal support, is able to use his awareness and focused attention, to facilitate flow of energy to different parts of his body—warming his hands or feet, and using grounding/gravity/out-breath to 'drain' the sensation of pain.

Third healing intention: To relieve pain, tightness in neck and shoulders and bring warmth to the body. He also wants to learn how to be calm, be in his body and have less anxiety. "I find that I am able to calm down and relieve my anxiety using the breath and grounding, centering and aligning." On the table his biofield is diffuse and buzzing but balanced from side to side, with a stringy flow to the ground. There is more energy around head and shoulders with hot spots on shoulders and back of neck. Hot spots are also noted off both hips and a cool thickness over his thighs. There is a tight empty sensation running from his sternum to his pelvis. Used an alignment technique to sweep the field with intention to calm and support the flow from head to feet. Encountered multiple layers of entangled energy above his torso where a dynamic mat slowly works loose with repeated sweeps of his field. With each sweep through the field stopping a bit at the 2nd and 4th chakra, his field visibly softens, his breathing became deeper, less clavicular and more soft- belly breathing. Move to the balancing the brain which takes some time to bring balance and flow and to stop the buzzing feeling. This is followed with the star treatment. Then I hold his ankles to ground him. His overall field increases flow from head to feet, no evidence of the buzzing edges noted pre scan. His biofield appears smooth and sense it is glowing. In response Jasper notes that his hands and feet are warm, as are his thighs. The pain has released from his back and shoulders. He appears quite excited: "I feel really good. I know this works I can really feel the difference". He says that others have noticed and commented on the difference in him as well. "The older men at the other AA I go to said I looked less stressed, I don't have as many lines on my face." Self-care: He will continue with grounding, centering and aligning.

Jasper arrives for his final healing session. He wants to talk through some of his experiences. He did not want to do table work. He shares his progress "This week I was really upset. I could feel myself going into depression. But I pre-empted the depression. I lay back down on my bed and worked to fill the whole room with peace, love and kindness. This was the first time I was able to hold that feeling throughout the whole room. I felt very good afterwards. I still feel good." We talk about holding space, in particular the type of space that he 'built' for himself in his room, how building it outside of ourselves takes a determined mind and a strong will, and how we can build this space from the inside out from our heart center. As we hold our heart center, we hold the space. We do an exercise reaffirming this method. In return he is able to go into his heart center and ground, center and align himself. He is excited and appears well grounded. We talk some more and then he thanks me for the time we spent together.

Jasper's quotes: "I was very skeptical at the beginning. I really knew it worked for me when I saw that I could relax my muscle tension which restricts my blood flow, and my hands and feet warmed. For me, the table work is okay, it was the work in the chairs that I found the most useful. This works so well with the cognitive behavior therapy they teach here. I have learned how to be quiet inside. Recently the Director of the recovery house called me into his office to say that he has really noticed the change in me, how calm I appear now, before I was really anxious a lot of the time." "I would like to take this out to other recovery homes." For Jasper it was about stillness and presence. He is going to use this in his life, especially at the recovery house.

These two gentle, guided, Integrative Energy Healing sets by practitioners (a nurse and a psychologist in this case) show how complex it is to assist clients returning to self—physical self—grounding into physical body. Clients related how they displaced their energy above their heads to energetically deplete the physical structure, especially to decrease their sense of grounding. This tactic freed them from truly feeling either the physical pain or tension in their body, or from sensing their own feelings, or both. Male clients also often experienced an imploded human energy field. That is, they had compressed— pushed energy into the central core of their body where it was stagnant but compact. Clients also often experienced disconnection from the present moment such that they had an uncanny ability to energetically disappear: Luke mentally disengaged noticeably and people even asked him if he was present, while Jasper 'numbed out' so he did not need to feel emotions or his aching body. In Jasper, the disconnect and resultant holding-in was extreme and expressed itself as Fibromyalgia and anxiety; the same pattern resulted in muscle pain in Luke, and in fear, depression, anxiety, physical discomfort, and boundary issues for other clients.

The extent to which clients used these mostly unconscious coping strategies related to how shielded or obliterated they had become and how removed they were from the physical, material source of their being. Practitioners carefully supported and encouraged return to the physical body via creating trust and rapport, and used breath, grounding techniques, and a wide range of subtle energy healing modalities with awareness dialogue. Their work was based on a full biofield assessment-evaluation that was dynamic in scope and always present to the moment (Lamb, 2010).

We felt Jasper was not fully ready to change his lifestyle as events unfolded; however, he was certainly ready to acknowledge other options and he gained a renewed sense of his power over his body, and thereby if he wished, over his addiction and cycling suicide attempts. He was sensitive to energy and capably noted how his physiology responded once his body had correct instructions and catalyst assistance from the practitioner. He used some of the integral strategies when he was on his own and saw the impact. However, this new information has to overcome the inertia-coded pathways and self-sabotage habits well ingrained in his lifestyle. Will he remember to breathe into his painful material-physical body when the migraines start or the Fibromyalgia pain increases? Will he remember to ground and align his heart with peacefulness when he next faces a wave of despair or depression, or frustration and anger? Will he remember, or will he return to the 'old-me' that knows drugs and suicide attempts palliate for a brief moment? This is for the future to tell.

In summary, when focusing on physical health, illness, and healing it is necessary to have awareness, even if minimally, of the material-physical, emotional-vital-physical, and mental- physical consciousness. Beyond this, an awareness of the soul's role in our lives and the other outer realms of consciousness brings further sophistication and yogic awareness. Accompanied with even rudimentary skills, this awareness provides for prompt healing responses when illness or dysfunctional forces threaten wellbeing.

The aim in healing is to develop the following: a depth of character that can sustain yogic abilities such that the fullness of our capacities can be accessed and utilized in a strong, quiet, and persistent manner; the willingness to nurture ourselves on many levels and dimensions; the ability to accept what comes (karmically or otherwise) as a means for growth and development; and agreement to sustain equanimity and faith moment-to-moment through all that life presents while still acting—manifesting the most sincere responses to all adversity.

We pause to consider Sri Aurobindo's words:

> ...The physical mind can be more easily opened and converted than the rest, but the vital-physical and the material-physical are obstinate. The old things are always recurring there without reason and by force of habit. Much of the vital-physical and most of the material are in the subconscience or depend on it. It needs a strong and sustained action to progress there. (Ghose, 2000b, p. 1445).

Yet, he reminds us, "...nothing can obstruct a quiet aspiration except one's own acquiescence in the inertia" (p. 1451). Let us turn now to a more synthetic view of the outer being from the lens of inner-being subliminal consciousness, particularly the subtle-body consciousness.

12
Subtle-Body Consciousness

It [the subliminal self] is connected with the small outer personality by certain centres of consciousness [chakras] of which we become aware by yoga. Only a little of the inner being escapes through these centres into the outer life, but that part is the best part of ourselves and responsible for our art, poetry, philosophy, ideals, religious aspirations, efforts at knowledge and perfection.
-Sri Aurobindo (Ghose, 2000b, p. 1165).

The subliminal self stands behind and supports the whole superficial man; it has in it a larger and more efficient mind behind the surface mind, a larger and more powerful vital behind the surface vital, a subtler and freer physical consciousness behind the surface bodily existence. And above them it opens to a higher superconscient as well as below them to the lower subconscient ranges.
-Sri Aurobindo (Ghose, 2000b, p. 1606).

Our human condition is positioned within vast realms that are challenging to understand; however, the ancient seers discovered a way to explain the beauty of our interconnection, and many cultures have their own narratives that explain human becoming. The Vedic seers saw the chakras and the *nadis* (ranging in number in the literature from 72,000 to 350,000) as formations of consciousness, force, energy, light, and information spread out at infinite angles of the causal, astral, subtle, and gross material levels—impacting the local and nonlocal aspects of human existence. In this chapter we address the basic aspects of the subtle inner-being linkages with the outer-being awareness.

Birthing yogic consciousness is one way of explaining inner awakening processes, because in this sense the chakra system is capable of unfolding consciousness, bringing more awareness to the outer being, and as we have seen, simultaneously initiating challenging inner processes for individuals. Many from the ancient Rishis forward have studied the chakra system, and Sri Aurobindo writes of this system in his journals, speaking about how he worked with different energy systems in his body and the Mother worked diligently to bring forth what they both call 'the mind of light' into the cellular consciousness (Ghose, 2000c).

However, from a broader perspective, Sri Aurobindo's yoga provides a synthesis: "the body is the bridge" (Satprem, see Enginger, 1992, p. 11) is a mainstay and motto of Integral yoga. In an ever unfolding manner, consciousness awakens in the physical, cellular, physiological, and genetic substance of our being. We must, Satprem admonishes, become more aware of the cell's power and the cell's knowledge, and discover the natural power and wisdom of the cells themselves through experiences. The Mother notes that this awareness will require a new type of perception, one that surpasses the access of ordinary consciousness. This access nurtures the subtle vibrations of a new consciousness in the cells, as the Mother firmly believed that lasting change comes at the cellular level (Alfassa, 1998).

Although lasting change requires a 'descent' into the body—a special descent of the spiritual-mind, thought-mind, and higher emotional-vital—it is nevertheless at the physical-mind level that real change will occur (Sri Aurobindo, see Ghose, 1996). This 'descent' requires us to live in the body and experience the body. One way to do so is to become sensitive to the coherence of the material-physical body while sensitizing ourselves to the subtle-energy body. There are many ways of doing so; however, India has provided much valuable literature based on ways of being, ways of living, chakras, breath work, and certain types of meditation—all designed to activate this deep inner awareness (White, 1990; Bakshi, 2004; Woodroffe, 2006).

The teachings support a paradoxical lesson: aspire with clarity, master your emotions, change your mind, and then your body will change (Satprem, see Enginger, 1992, p. 79). Hence, to change your body you must quieten your mind, all of them—that is, thought-mind, emotional-mind, sensory-mind, and physical- mind. Nevertheless, it takes the mind to understand the process. It takes a wisdom-based aspiration, rejection, and surrender—to the exact degree required—to reach deep into the cellular structures and encode for change.

The Mother suggests that with each dis-order, the secret to healing in the best way possible lies with a few cells. And the way to find these key cells is to use a biofield subtle-energy vibrational technique that requires an understanding of how subtle energy works within the inner being. Once these cells are found, the position of consciousness can be changed (Satprem, see Enginger, 1992, p. 94). This highly sophisticated process, she says, is designed to remove falsehood and bring a true calm, an inner light, and a will-to-health. Use the spiritual-mind and higher-emotional-vital aspects to embrace a vibration of Truth; in other words, be sensitive enough at this very micro-subtle level to identify a vibration of falsehood and to replace it with a vibration of Truth (Alfassa, 1998). With the vibration of Truth— sensed as a heartfelt, peaceful coherence and spaciousness— there must be no contraction, no reaction, and no inner refusal, only surrender to the vastness of peaceful coherent vibrations. The subconscient with its negative override must not be allowed to interfere, hence the need for thought-mind and an inspired higher order vital-emotional consent. This consent allows the consciousness of the cells to change, creating a new reality. (Satprem, see Enginger, 1992). There has been a change in the position of consciousness, an inner multidimensional attitude change: a new vibrational attunement in the stuff of consciousness.

Sri Aurobindo discusses one view of this multidimensional change process; his explanation is detailed, but the process is complex.

> The sensation in the spine and on both sides of it is a sign of the awakening of the Kundalini Power. It is felt as a descending and an ascending current. There are two main nerve-channels for the currents, one on each side of the central channel in the spine. The descending current is the energy from the above coming down to touch the sleeping Power in the lowest nerve centre at the bottom of the spine; the ascending current is the release of the energy going up from the awakened Kundalini. This movement as it proceeds opens all six centres of the subtle nervous system and by the opening one escapes from the limitations of the surface consciousness bound to the gross body and great ranges of experiences proper to the subliminal self, mental, vital, subtle physical are shown to the sadhak. When the Kundalini meets the higher Consciousness as it ascends through the summit of the head, there is an opening of the higher superconscient reaches above the normal mind...in our yoga it is not necessary to go through the systematized method. It takes place spontaneously according to the need and by the force of the aspiration. As soon as there is an opening the Divine Power descends and conducts the necessary working, does what is needed, each thing in its own time, and the yogic Consciousness begins to be born in the sadhak. (Ghose, 2000b, pp. 1147-1148).

The activities of the central channel (or sushumna channel) are instrumental in providing the force and consciousness for all change, and it is personal *tapasaya*—ongoing diligent purification—that Sri Aurobindo believes refines the Consciousness in its multimodal forms as force, power, energy, light and information which actually creates the evolutionary changes (Ghose, 2000b). His teachings suggest that the heart and higher mind openings are primary, and that this Kundalini force is also "above our head as the Divine Force—not there coiled up, involved and asleep, but awake, scient, potent, extended, wide; it is there waiting for manifestation and to this Force we have to open ourselves..." (Ghose, 2006, p. 153).

There is much still to be learned in the area of biofield and yogic science. Sri Aurobindo, scholar that he was, encouraged the development of ideas over time and across cultures.

What follows is my rebirth story rendition generally congruent with Integral yoga that explains how the central channel, nadis, chakras and auric field interact in the subtle body consciousness: the Return.

Destiny calls—a rebirth is imminent. Absolute Consciousness, Force, Energy, Light, and Information start to congeal at the most subtle, causal level of universal development. This process is a mystery, and it is mystical. However, quantum, or nonlocal waves of possibility or seeds of Consciousness, Force, Energy, Light, and Information now becoming Relative create a substance and a formation, presenting opportunities for the consciousness to descend; as this Relative consciousness builds, conception occurs. Consciousness in-the-formation-of-energy crystallizing initiates the process, and consciousness in-the-formation-of-matter for this new birth initiates at conception.

This massive creative force of consciousness is guided by the gunas, sattwa, rajas, and tamas energy flows with their calm, dynamic, and stabilizing forces turned inward. Further, the gunas in downward causality create vibratory bandwidths of causal, astral, and subtle energy symbollically called the Five Elements: Space or Ether, Air, Fire, Water, and Earth. The elements are a metaphor: each of the elements linked into or creating the nadis—infinitely tiny

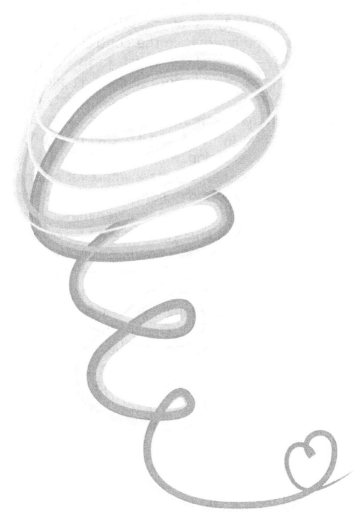

The Return

strings of energy that are sources for the infinite gradients of energy required as astral and subtle bodies develop—has ideological characteristics that fit the conceptual rendition of these complex bandwidths of multidimensional energy. The interweaving of the gunas with the elements and nadis creates the template for the formation of the embryo. This interweaving creates the central channel (technically the sushumna, ida, pingala, and even more subtle channels).

Soon, combinations of causal, astral, and subtle consciousness-force building in the central channel create points of energy—the chakras—which form the auric field and the major nerve plexus, both supporting and sustaining further development. These energy focal points or chakras have been called the seven 'major chakras'. They are major transducers of energy, and create the bridge between energy and matter, emotion, and thought, spirit and place. There are chakras or energy centers wherever a bone meets a bone and at all major and minor nerve centers; however, the literature tends to focus on the seven major chakras, or vortexes of empowered energy, each with its own complex role in the development and ongoing functioning of the body, emotions, mind, and spirit.

Once the energy, in power and impetus, elements, and gunas has congealed enough, etheric substance creates cells that form and multiply. The central channel sustains and supports the development of the embryo and fetus according to both designated genetic patterns from family heritage, environmental influences, and karmic aspects—Information carried within the consciousness itself.

Chakras form from the crown down, seventh to first. The crown chakra is formed first, as the fetus has a stronger connection with the spiritual realms, the forces of beauty and light that set the destiny-call, than to the earth-based world. Next to form is the ajna or sixth chakra at the brow level, followed by the fifth chakra at the throat and the fourth chakra at the heart level, third at the solar plexus, second in the middle of the lower abdomen, and the first chakra in the perineal area, connected to earth energy and the child's role here on the planet.

The auric field co-forms along with the chakras, and auric dimensions are co-located and interpenetrated within the chakras, both empowered by the central channel. While composed of many-dimensional layers, the aura or human energy field has five commonly identified layers: *anandamaya kosha* or bliss body—place of illumined

Unity; *vijnanamaya kosha*, or intelligence layer—home of ideals and higher abstract ideas, known as the causal layer; *manomaya kosha* or mind substance layer—place of many dimensional thought forms, known as the mental layer; *pranamaya kosha* or life force and emotional layer—dynamic, rajasic and feeling-toned with many dimensional desires and sensations, known as the astral layer; and the most dense, annamaya kosha, or most physical layer built from food molecules—closely blueprints the physical body, known as the subtle layer. Each layer has its unique 'consciousness- conditioned' role with force, energy, light, and information simultaneously presenting parallel dimensions that function in unity when there is inner coherence.

Accessing higher energies and lower energies in infinite and nonlocal ranges, the central channel or *sushumna* supporting the seven major chakras and the auric field sustains the ongoing development of genetic, molecular, biochemical, physiological, and biological development as tissues are formed and align for specific functions. The central channel also supports the nonmaterial aspects of growth and development—as the emotional-vital body forms, the mental body, and of course the more subtle, inner-being nature with the innermost being or soul actively guiding this new birth.

Amazingly, consciousness translates and transduces in gradient packages to form resonances the body can use at the microatomic and cellular levels, developing for example the neurotransmitters, hormones, and all the tissues. Moreover, the amazing transductions of energy co-create with matter, along with the emotional, mental, and spiritual aspects unique to the human experience. We are energetic beings blessed with infinite dimensions of consciousness, vibrating resonances of light, multiple layers of information, co-creating in ways we still cannot fathom within the great universal order as it impacts this one extended moment: this lifetime.

We are biochemical, neurologic, emotional, mental, and spiritual beings, we are electric, and electromagnetic beings, we connect to infinite ranges of consciousness and energy simplified into the designations subtle, astral, causal and bliss; our physiology and our psychology is as spiritual as it is material; it is based on the blueprints of Consciousness, Force, Energy, Light, and Information. What initiates this subtle connection between energy and matter is still a mystery.

At this time, we remain at the meta level with consciousness, force, light, and information as the primary causative factor in co-creation and the particle-wave the primary force engaging with Nature's design, interwoven with the Divine decree to 'return'. Consciousness provides the force and information, and Nature provides the template for structures ranging from gross to subtle. The multiple nadis— exceedingly tiny micro-channels of energy—support and sustain the energy-body, ensuring that physiological processes maintain their capacity and prescribed functions.

When the energy system is compromised, health is impacted. It is believed that chronic illnesses show first in the energy system or biofield, and only secondly in the physiology or gross matter. However, all illness or dis-ease impacts the whole state-of-being (physical, emotional-vital, mental, and spiritual), as well as the multidimensional energy of the inner and outer being.

Sri Aurobindo (Ghose, 2004) used the chakras in his yoga but he did not see them as a main feature; in this chapter, we view his Integral yoga configuration but add congruent nuances from my research and the literature. The chakras are subtle, invisible to the ordinary vision, present in the inner being consciousness, and visible to extended vision, or high sense perception, as vortexes or wheels of light. Each chakra is associated with a nerve plexus and is influenced by complex bandwidths of consciousness from the physiology—that is, from gross matter, emotional reactions, responses, and a whole range of thought associated with the outer being. Additionally and to a much higher degree, the inner being and innermost being influences subtle energy connections and physiology; moreover, the individual environmental and external   environmental influences have impact (Dalal, 2007).

The following table presents the seven major chakras and their characteristics. These chakras comprise the inner being, composed of the supraconscient, subconscient, inconscient, and circumconscient. Together, the inner being elements compose the outer being, which is influenced from all aspects of the outer and inner being.

Chakras and Characteristics

CHAKRA	CHARACTERISTICS
CHAKRA 7: Sahasradala GLAND: Pineal SYSTEM: Central Nervous	INFLUENCE FROM: higher mind, illumined and intuitive mind, opens to Brahman—infinite consciousness LINKED TO: identification, higher understanding, and direct knowing ELEMENT: Beyond elements—Bliss
CHAKRA 6: Ajna GLAND: Pituitary SYSTEM: Autonomic Nervous	INFLUENCE FROM: higher mind, spiritual-mind, with inner will and inner vision, thought-mind LINKED TO: Ideals of Yogic consciousness, clarity ELEMENT: Beyond elements—Light

Chakra	Characteristics
Chakra 5: Visuddha Gland: Thyroid System: Respiratory Plexus: Thyroid	Influence from: thought-mind, mechanical or material- mind, emotional-vital-mind, and the higher-vital Linked to: Externalized expression, creativity, communication, and purification Element: Ether/Space
Chakra 4: Anahata Soul-Access: Chaitya Purusha Gland: Thymus System: Circulatory Plexus: Cardiac	Influence from: emotional-vital-mind, higher-vital Access to inner heart, soul or psychic being consciousness Linked to: Higher emotions, lower emotions, egoic compassion, and Service Element: Air
Chakra 3: Manipura Gland: Pancreas System: Digestive Plexus: Solar	Influence from: emotional-vital-mind, higher-vital and emotional-vital Linked to: Aspects of action, egoic mastery, larger desire- based movements Element: Fire

CHAKRA	CHARACTERISTICS
CHAKRA 2: Svadhistana GLAND: Ovaries and Testes SYSTEM: Reproductive PLEXUS: Pelvic	INFLUENCE FROM: physical-mind, lower emotional-vital, emotional-vital-physical LINKED TO: Emotional relationships and smaller desires ELEMENT: Water
CHAKRA 1: Muladhara GLAND: Adrenal SYSTEM: Excretory and skeletal PLEXUS: Coccyx/sacral	INFLUENCE FROM: material- physical, lower emotional- vital, physical-vital- emotional, mental-physical LINKED TO: Physical consciousness, primal instinctual reactions, need- based emotions, and a sense of safety ELEMENT: Earth

Of the many chakras throughout the energy body system, seven are featured here. Sri Aurobindo's system is utilized along with additional information on the glands, nerve plexus, systems impacted, and element (Dalal, 2007; Johari, 2000).

The seventh or *Sahasradala* chakra brings influence from the higher mind, illumined and intuitive mind and opens to infinite consciousness—Brahman. It is linked to identification or direct knowing and higher understanding, and influences the pineal gland and Central Nervous System. Its focus is Bliss states, beyond the five elements.

The *Ajna*, or sixth chakra also receives influences from the higher mind, spiritual-mind, thought-mind and connects with inner will and inner vision. It is linked to ideas of yogic consciousness and clarity, and is also beyond elements and has affinity with Light. It influences the pituitary gland and Autonomic Nervous System.

The *Visuddha* or fifth chakra brings influence from thought-mind, mechanical or material-mind, emotional-vital mind, and the higher-vital. It is linked to externalized expression and creativity, communication, and a desire for purification, and influences the thyroid gland, thyroid plexus, and Respiratory system. It resonates to the element Space or Ether.

The *Anahata* or fourth chakra brings influence from the emotional-vital-mind and higher-vital, and when appropriately open, there is access to the inner heart, soul, or psychic being consciousness. It is linked to higher emotions such as love, joy, forgiveness, and compassion, and lower emotions such as sorrow and hatred, as well as to egoic compassion and to Service for higher and egoic reasons. It resonates to the element Air. When there is a conscious soul connection, it is termed access to the Chaitya Purusha. The fourth chakra influences the thymus gland, cardiac, and Circulatory system.

The *Manipura* or third chakra brings influence from the emotional-vital-mind and higher-vital. It is linked to aspects of action, egoic mastery, and larger desire-based movements. It resonates to the element Fire.

The *Svadhistana* or second chakra receives influence from the physical-mind, lower emotional-vital, and emotional-vital-physical. It is linked to emotional relationships and smaller desires, and resonates to the element Water.

The *Muladhara* or first chakra receives influence from the material-physical, lower emotional-vital, and physical-vital emotional. It is linked to physical consciousness, cellular consciousness, primal instinctual reactions, need-based emotions, and a sense of safety. It resonates with the element Earth. (More detail on chakras is readily available in other literature, less so in Integral yoga literature).

Sri Aurobindo noted that the seventh, sixth, and fifth chakras are more mental in their utilization of consciousness; the fourth, third, and second are more emotional; and the first chakra is more directly related to the physical and subsconscient. However, the subtle inner being consciousness interacts with all levels of the being— outer and inner being. Immediate contact is made via the micro-nadi system, the chakra system, and the central channel that sustains them, as well as the other micro and macro channel systems and the biofield system.

Note the chakra system in the image:

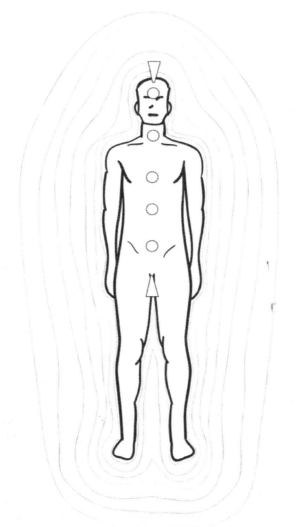

Chakras with Auric Field

Surrounding it is the auric field, or biofield, sometimes called the human energy field or personal circumconscient immersed in the environmental circumconscient. In essence, this field has infinite dimensional connections; however, to make the context manageable it is associated here with the classic seven chakras. The chakras are rooted into the *central channel* or the *kundalini channel* consisting of the *ida, pingala*, and *sushumna nadis*. These are all at the subtle level, non-visible to ordinary site. They intersect with the infinite nonlocal aspects of consciousness—here is where the gross, subtle, astral, and causal intersect.

Note the seven chakras situated in the central channel that runs along the spinal column within the subtle body—with their concentric spiralling, these chakras develop the outer levels of the auric field. Each of these levels is mirrored internally at both a micro- and macro-level within every cell. That is, each cell of our 100 million cells has the potential for consciousness at all seven vibratory levels (and more.)

The nervous envelope or auric biofield can support, protect, and sustain a person when it is intact. This biofield consists of subtle energy that surrounds the body creating a force field. When fully charged, it repels bacteria, viruses, and intrusive attacks; if it is fractured, thin, weak, fragile, or torn, this field cannot protect and adverse forces may enter through it to the body-consciousness, with cellular pathology following.

Prior to the establishment of disease, the Mother (Alfassa, 2006) says, if individuals are receptive enough they will recognize when a disharmonious presence has access to the body-consciousness. She describes a four-step process of active protection presented here as the *Yogic Reharmonization Process* (see table below). First, instantly reject the negative or hostile force and enhance the protective auric biofield; second, over a few minutes scan the biofield, seal all openings, and dissolve any sense of the negative force that has gained entry into the biofield;

third, place a clear and direct divine Force on the areas of discomfort where the force has gained access and maintain this steadfastly for several hours; fourth, continue the work (potentially for days) to reduce symptoms and clear pathology.

The process involves focusing the Force of peace, stillness, and divine Power—pushing and pressing it into the cells carrying the dysfunctional energies. In these practices the Mother suggests that individuals call on the following: the inner wiser consciousness, the intuitive awareness held in the subliminal consciousness; the soul; and, in general, the higher vital and mental spiritual aspects of consciousness, including the use of prayer.

Sri Aurobino offers this reminder:

> All illnesses pass through the nervous or vital-physical sheath of the subtle consciousness and subtle body before they enter the physical (Ghose, 1998, p. 236).

Use of: inner wiser consciousness, the soul, higher vital, mental spiritual aspects of consciousness + prayer.

Yogic Reharmonization Process

Step	Immediate action	Ongoing action
One	Instantly reject negative force.	Using breath and intention, strengthen the auric biofield.
Two	Scan the biofield, seal all openings in the auric biofield.	Dissolve any negative forces that have gained entry. Recharge the auric biofield. Identify remaining areas of disharmony— dissolve and release disruptions.

Step	Immediate action	Ongoing action
Three	If forces have gained access: Place Peace, Calm, and Light on the target areas.	Maintain a concentrated-focus of Peace, Calm, and Light on areas of disruption for several hours.
Four	If disorder sets in: Continue placing Peace, Calm, and Light on the area or into targeted cells.	Holding steadfast focus, press the Peace, Calm, and Light into the targeted area and cellular structures—for days if necessary.

The specific strategies outlined by Sri Aurobindo and the Mother are diverse and vary for each individual; they stress the uniqueness of each person. However, Sri Aurobindo and the Mother both focus on the following recommendations for building health (Alfassa, 1998; Ghose & Alfassa, 2006).

• Develop an inward consciousness by learning to sense the force of division or slight uneasiness as it comes toward you;

• Reinforce the nervous envelope or auric biofield when it is depleted, and insert a wall of quiet, peaceful vibration when required;

• Notice symptoms while they are still subtle or in the subtle physical, and dissipate them;

• Cut off the connection to pain and widen oneself to embrace the light;

• Turn the consciousness upward via aspiration, invocation, and prayer, and call on the divine Power;

• Face fear and dissolve fear;

• Turn attention elsewhere and refuse to let the condition become important;

• Infuse confidence in all aspects of the physical, emotional-vital, and mental;

• Develop a conscious contact with peace—a dynamic peace—by drawing peace into the self, into the solar plexus, and then directing it to the symptom area;

• Throw out all attacking forces;
• Open high sense perception as many senses are asleep;
• Withdraw the body's consent and separate inner consciousness from outer or body-consciousness such that it is not 'you' who is ill—sense behind material creation to complete peaceful immobility;
• Set in action the inner power of the physical, vital, and mental subliminal and psychic consciousness;
• And, access a deep and pure faith.

Healing requires all of the above in addition to the power of the Force—the willingness, aspiration, intention, and integrity of the instrument. This knowledge is to be used as an adjunct for self-care, in conjunction with professional assistance when required. Responsible professional guidance and personal responsibility go hand in hand.

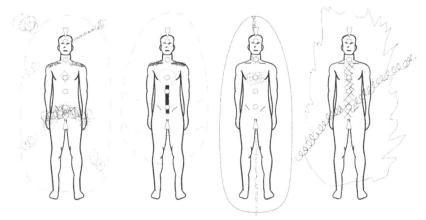

Biofield Disruption

The images above are sketches drawn from the research that depict how the auric biofield (sometimes called the human energy field) responds to adverse influence. In many cases, at the start of the session the research participants could scan their own biofield and note areas of disruption. After the practitioners had worked with them using an awareness-based dialogue and specific biofield-healing techniques, differences could be noted— not only in the biofield but also in the participant's overall emotional tone and mental clarity. The clients experiential 'noticing', with a witness consciousness able to understand, brought hope and renewed faith in the individual's own ability to heal. This experience encouraged resilience and provided an impetus for ongoing learning, and could initiate further efforts in self-mastery—of course, all within the level of 'readiness' unique to that individual and available to all.

The next chapter presents Julia's story, a delightful, thoughtful, and highly sensitive sharing of her process of human becoming to where she is at this time. Her story shows how a deeper, broader, and witness-based understanding can make a difference—and change a life.

13
JULIA'S STORY

...there is a consciousness much wider, more
luminous, more in possession of itself and things
than that which wakes upon our surface and is the
percipient of our daily hours; that is our inner being,
and it is this we must regard as our subliminal self
and set apart the subconscient as an inferior, a
lowest occult province of our nature.
-Sri Aurobindo (Ghose, 2000c, p. 557).

When Julia (pseudonym), a graduate of the Integrative
Energy Healing program submitted her final reflection
paper she provided a fine example of the poignantly lived
processes embraced in Sri Aurobindo's Integral yoga. She
speaks to many of the integral processes and the struggles
that occur between the inner and outer being. She shares
how war zone consciousness can overtake, and even so she
again touches the inner wisdom, soul-consciousness that
was there with her as a child. After reading her paper I
asked her if she would expand it some and be willing to
share her deepening healing process with others. She
agreed. Here is her story.

As a small child, I inhabited a magical, protected
realm, floating through the days in a dreamy, open state
where I felt secure and whole, with a natural sense of
where I had come from and where I belonged. My early life
unfolded against a rich tapestry of tales about the daily
lives of an industrious group of people who had settled the
depopulated Danubian Plain in Eastern Europe as these lands
were reclaimed from the receding Turkish empire. It was
told how, as part of a great colonization scheme launched
by the Austrian Imperial Council in the seventeenth century,
my ancestors had set forth in specially designed barges
which they dismantled and turned into roof rafters upon

their arrival. The pioneers' mission had been to transform the vacated wastelands into rich farmlands; in time, their labors turned this area into a bread basket for the entire region. I felt proud to be an inheritor of such bravery and resourcefulness.

Though not from Germany, my resourceful people who had lived peacefully among their neighbours for centuries were stripped of their civil rights and their property in the aftermath of WWII, due to their predominantly German ethnic origin. They were subjected to mass expulsions, and many who stayed were annihilated. All four of my father's grandparents, feeling too old to accompany their neighbours on the difficult journey to freedom, succumbed to the genocide in starvation camps close to where they had lived.

When the war was ending, my father, just in his late teens, was dragged off for three years to a forced labor camp in the coal mines of Russia. On his return he was wounded as he took much needed food from a farmer's field. He eventually recovered and gained a valued skill.

My mother's family walked with their neighbours across the rutted roads of three countries, leaving behind their self- sustaining farm and taking only what fit in their wagon. Often pushing to help their two remaining farm horses along the muddy way, stopping only to eat or to sleep in the barns or haystacks of kindly farmers, they arrived eventually in a land that was strange to them. After seven years spent in that country which never became home, my mother's family were the first from their host village to leave for Canada, as soon as they learned of this opportunity.

All these things I knew of, though I had no way of understanding them within a broader context; I simply took them in stride, perhaps because the adults tended to leave out the parts about their pain. I sometimes wondered why no one apart from my relatives and their friends appeared to know of 'my people'. I know now that the events which befell them have not been made widely known, and the reasons why their history is not taught in schools. Eventually both my father and mother arrived, married, started a family, and then immigrated to Canada.

I understood very early how, just as my family had gifted me with a heritage of exploring new frontiers, so must my life be an exploration into the unknown. On our arrival, my parents had not yet mastered the new language, and I was left to interpret many things for myself. Although I did not know how to speak English when I first went to kindergarten, I understood most of what went on through some mysterious process of osmosis; I remember feeling baffled by others' inability to understand me

As time went on, I began to notice darker threads weaving through the fabric of our lives. Given their background, my parents were especially careful to protect us from the dangers and cruelty immigrant families sometimes encounter. On occasion, I did not understand my father's seemingly disproportionate reactions to what I thought of as innocent events. Sometimes I did not understand why I was being scolded when I believed I had used good judgement; from my perspective, my father had clearly misinterpreted the situation by erupting as though there had been a great danger. How could I have even begun to guess at the inner turmoil he was hiding, even from himself?

Unfolding

It began a very long time ago, though I did not notice it then. Perhaps it was when I was a baby, or a child, or when I was becoming a woman. It surfaced in my teen years as a feeling of un-ease; eventually, it felt like dis-ease. I did not feel safe, though I could not name my fear at the time.

I had been an open-minded, intuitive child, easily reaching out to others when I perceived them to be in distress, yet my awareness of the emotions of those close to me often left me confused—their illogical behaviors often appeared to deny the reality of what I was sensing. I did not know then that the soft boundaries—so common in an empathic child struggling to be understood in an environment characterized by constricted interrelationships—were also fertile ground for the development of a distorted sense of 'place' in the world. As I became more confused between what was mine and what was someone else's, I began to feel a disproportionate burden of responsibility for others' behaviors as well as for their concealed distress, and gradually became confused about my own identity. As I grew, I found my own version of inner balance: walking a fine line between the conflicting messages I was receiving from my environment, the role-playing I felt was required of me, and my inner inclination to spin, dance, float, and laugh with joy. Thus, I became adept at realigning with my inner truth in private, for little fragments of time, holding onto the fragile thread that kept a deeper part of me connected with the relative sanity of my inner knowing.

As I entered the world more, I tried finding creative solutions to the puzzle of life, often blindly— straining to hear the guidance of a tiny, fading voice within and becoming increasingly distressed by the harsh, discordant noise bearing down on me from 'outside'. I became less able to distinguish between inner truth and a story I'd invented. Many mistakes, blind alleys, wrong turns, and manifestations of outer conflict and its resulting inner struggle occurred in my world as I trusted myself less and less.

I began to rebel inside, insisting on following a barely discernable path, preferring to move forward with faith in the unknown rather than follow a prescribed path I could not believe in. My sense of what was real became confused as I struggled to make sense of my increasingly baffling life in an increasingly complicated world. I did not know at the time that it would be many, many years before I could begin to understand how this bafflement concerned much more than the resolution of an inner tension—it was, in fact, about survival.

Over the course of years, illogical beliefs and misconceptions manifested regarding my personal identity and the relative 'place' of that identity within a greater universe. The structure of my inner reality formed around a conviction that I was at fault, to blame, at the mercy of outside forces more powerful than myself; that I was not 'allowed' to shine, to let my inner brilliance be seen on the outside; and that my insight, inner wisdom, and natural intuition must remain hidden as I privately struggled with contradictions between what I 'knew' to be true and what I was supposed to accept as true. I began to feel a vague sense that something was 'wrong' perhaps a year or two before I moved into puberty, but was unable to quite put my finger on what it was.

When I was about 15, I went out one evening to a campfire with a friend and some boys she knew. My parents had given their permission, and I assumed all was well. As I arrived back home, the floor was abruptly pulled out from under me and my world as I knew it came crashing down. I went into shock as I felt myself assaulted by a verbal battering for which I could find no sense or reason. Sometime later, when the torrent of enraged words finally stopped slicing into me and I had still not been allowed to speak, I was reeling with a confusion so intense I began alternating between agony and complete dissociation as I felt the life I had known quietly slipping away. I truly did not know what had gone wrong (and we never discussed it since). Throughout the next day, I was unable to stop crying—a deep, anguished, forlorn crying—and after that I went numb inside. In my disoriented state, I no longer felt like I belonged anywhere.

For a very long time, I was unable to piece together what could possibly have caused this violation of my identity, nor was I able to determine the reason for such intense rage toward me, but from that night forward, I was no longer the same person inside. It took some time to understand that it was I who had shattered, while my world continued as it had been. I gradually began to feel my sense of reality becoming distorted as I tried to piece back together what now felt violently torn apart. I had gone from being a more or less normal—though somewhat insecure and naïve—inquisitive teenager that afternoon, to a traumatized, confused, fragmented wreck by midnight, and did not understand why.

Though I tried hard to continue with my life in the usual way, I gradually began to experience physical and psychological symptoms of severe anxiety, no longer feeling comfortable in my own skin, my home, or in my world. I often felt distracted and had difficulty focussing. I felt tight bands around my head as I sat at my desk trying to take in what the teacher was saying. I began to suffer from digestive distress and experienced great difficulty falling asleep.

I began to behave differently, knowing that it didn't matter what I did—since in my interpretation, I had been informed unequivocally that I was an utter failure regardless of what I did or didn't do. I would skip classes and spend the time sitting by a wall behind the school, smoking and writing dark poetry, obsessively striving to find the exact way to express what was trying to translate itself from the part of my consciousness where there are no words. There were no longer any clear lines on the map of my life by which I could orient myself, and the map was irretrievably dissolving into a strange, shapeless blur.

My inner distress and sense of alienation continued to expand until, by my late teens, the growing tension caused by a multitude of conflicting messages and contradictions in logic (not to mention the ravaging shocks of perceived betrayal and psychological violation) began to disrupt the continuity of my consciousness until eventually it propelled me toward a breakdown. In my desperation to feel through the numbness, I started cutting myself, and once, casually while at school, overdosed myself with antidepressants I had 'obtained'. The medical 'intervention' I received left me even more distressed. I moved out of the family home once I had completed high school. Despite this attempt to free myself from the confusing elements I had been experiencing while living there, in my obsession to understand the 'truth' I had essentially stopped sleeping for so long—painting all night instead—that the veils between states of consciousness grew thin. Finally, I lost my bearings, dreaming while awake, hallucinating, 'racing' with adrenaline, my speech coming out in strange, overlapping expression.

The treatment I received then felt harsh and inappropriate to what I felt I needed. Rather than being asked about what I was experiencing, I was labelled, drugged once again, and essentially ignored for several weeks, having emphatically refused the shock therapy which appeared to be the primary treatment administered in that facility. I felt like I was being punished, and instead of having received meaningful help, a new layer of trauma had been added. I tried to patch myself back together despite these baffling ministrations by misguided 'experts', and a year later, I sought and received some more enlightened, gentler help. This created somewhat of a shift in my previous sense of 'condemnation' yet, had I understood then how long and hard the journey ahead of me would be, I might not have found the strength to continue. I struggled for years with paranoia, fearing that if my inner turmoil were to be discovered or if I were to take a serious misstep, I would be shunned or once again controlled by forces greater than myself.

I pushed myself through university, defying the conventions that appeared to encourage boys but not girls (or at least not me) to pursue their intellectual aspirations. In my interpretation, women were expected to be supported by a man, with possibly a side career to help maintain the household. While it was anticipated that I would work, I perceived no indication that I was expected to accomplish anything particularly noteworthy; yet simultaneously, I was required to excel at my tasks and in school, never quite able to meet the ambiguous standard reflected in my father's eyes.

My desire had been to develop my natural artistic abilities, yet I was unable to find career guidance that was meaningful to me. Still reeling inside and feeling splintered from unresolved inner tensions, I persevered relentlessly though blindly and with no clear concept of where I was headed. I was on a mission and resolved to keep going until I achieved it, certain that I would discover my destination as I proceeded.

After one particularly stressful experience, I began to experience a chronic state of hyper-vigilance, my anxiety beginning to reach almost intolerable levels at times. I began struggling with physical distress in the form of Irritable Bowel Syndrome, extreme menstrual cramping, and heart palpitations.

I did not inform my family of this experience for fear of unsettling them. I had no way of knowing how individuals would react, and wasn't willing to risk this unknown. Had I told them, I may have received some compassion, but as it was, the barrage of disparaging comments from my father were increasing as his own inner process evolved, and instead of being able to heal, I simply felt battered. It was around this time that I began to suspect he had suffered some severe trauma in his life which had not healed. However, not having healed sufficiently myself, and— unknowingly at the time—going through my own version of what I now recognize as Post-Traumatic Stress Disorder, I was unable to reconcile these psychological attacks despite the compassion I felt for him.

Often floundering and having to regroup, I finally graduated seven years later with a degree I did not feel able to utilize. I decided I must make my living in a more practical way, and thankfully had been working throughout my studies at the university to support myself and pay tuition. I was able to easily turn this experience into a progression of full time jobs in which I developed increasingly accomplished skills and discovered abilities I had never guessed at. In short, I excelled at my work and found opportunities to take on progressively higher levels of responsibility. While striving to incorporate creativity into my approach to tasks, I stretched my capacity for left-brain focus, meanwhile beginning to recognize my previous lack of balance characterized by right-brain dominance. Thus I inadvertently began building a career path around a pattern recognizable to me as a succession of what I thought of as "creative missions."

In time, I found myself working for a dynamic company that gave me the opportunity to create my own position. Driven by an inner vision, I stretched my left brain abilities along with my level of responsibility further than I ever had, my efforts eventually contributing substantially to their bottom line. Meanwhile, I was working on the side in an artistic endeavor as a way of achieving better balance in which my right brain was being exercised.

During this time, I was encountering situations in which I found myself being verbally attacked by certain people. This pattern had begun to show up prior to this, though at the time I had considered the events as isolated incidents. In some manner I couldn't identify, I appeared to be attracting verbal assaults from a successive string of aggressive people. I found this puzzling, given that everyone else including the upper management appeared to appreciate my approach and I was enjoying a high level of success in team-oriented problem solving. The intensity of these exchanges increased as I refused to topple, and needless to say, this kind of triggering resulted in inner distress beyond the scope of the actual situation. While I recognized that something within me was pulling out these hostile behaviors in particular individuals, I somehow wasn't able to stop the pattern.

Slowly I became aware of the deeper resonance with older trauma that these episodes elicited in me, and came to look at it as an inner lesson in learning how to detach myself from a sense of responsibility for another's hostile behavior. I still encounter situations occasionally in which another tries to take advantage or bully me, but once I recognize and process the pattern, I'm finding it easier to stand up for myself in ways that actually bring about a positive change in the other's behavior toward me.

Much later, I decided to begin re-exploring my more natural artistic and holistic inclinations. I found myself enrolled and on the road to learning about energy healing, believing I had finally given myself permission to embark upon a journey into the intriguing world of my inner longing, choosing to have faith in my ability to sustain myself somehow.

What has occurred for me during this time of reorientation was unexpected. I had worked so hard through all those intervening years on resolving my old hurts—taking workshops, doing reflective journaling, visiting holistic practitioners, practicing yoga—that I had been convinced I had already been healing myself quite effectively.

My journey home

I began to understand that feeling safe is a much broader and deeper subject than I had ever before recognized. As I had been witnessing my own inner process, many truths have been unveiled that were previously shadowed, disguised, and hidden within, or behind, habituated thought, emotion, and physical, behavioral, and relational patterns. Now, as I shine my light of understanding into the dark corners , yet more unhealed fragments of my crouching, trembling self emerged, waiting— waiting to be recognized and released from their splintered condition and to rejoin the whole of who I Am.

I learned about witnessing and, for me, witnessing began with the intention to witness. As though awaiting even the slightest opportunity to come forth out of hiding, layer upon layer of buried patterns of belief, clusters of emotion, and loops of thought began to flow out; they emerged through the cracks now opening in the surface of the shell around a seemingly bottomless chasm deep within, unfolding to release their precious contents into the light of my consciousness for acknowledgement and release.

Most often, thoughts bubbled up into the relatively clear pool of my waking mind, where dreaming was done and the gears of linear thought had not yet begun their endless churning. They came as echoes of experience, often in the form of the actual 'felt' emotions that had accompanied long ago trauma. For so long I had been aware of these emotions primarily as remembrances filtered through the rational thought process —that is, I 'knew' of the feelings conceptually but was not able to remember the actual somatic experience of them. In essence, I appear to have suspended these emotions at the point of original impact, unable for many years to process them to conclusion. The vague sense of being 'dampened' and 'depressed' had become a familiar undercurrent, perhaps a comfort zone. Now, I began feeling these undercurrents ripple through my body and conscious awareness unexpectedly: sudden waves of emotion or physical sensations that cleansed and released the trapped energy as it surged through and I was finally able to name it. I recognized anxiety, terror, humiliation, betrayal, violation, unshed grief, a feeling of being (psychologically) smashed to bits, crushed, clamped down, emotionally strangled, and so forth.

As these experiences were recognized, felt, and released, insight occurred spontaneously — sometimes simultaneously and sometimes a little later. At times, a sudden understanding popped forth as I was drinking my morning tea, driving to work, or walking along the river path. As the connections between prior events and present behavioral patterns clicked into place in my conscious awareness, I began to recognize the overwhelming effect that these perceived and actual assaults had produced in my sensitive energy field. I perceived the repercussions that had developed over time in my physical state and the thought loops cycling endlessly through my waking mind, coloring my rational process.

I witnessed the ways in which I had been repressing my own clarity of perception, not only of present reality but also of the devastating after-effects of former insults and violations. I recognized my pattern of deflecting direct awareness, substituting it almost instantly with a reinterpretation that seemed more suitable to the model I had created for surviving in the world. In essence, I was habitually flipping the truth over and replacing it with a 'suitable lie' as a way of explaining the world—and my own discomfort. I had begun to believe the lies I was telling myself, attributing these effects to some mysterious flaw within. I would obsess about what inner fault in me could have caused another to behave in a certain way toward me, while compulsively sabotaging my health or my efforts to build effective structures in my life. At other times, I would create a heroic story in which I was a warrior fighting for a cause, or a benevolent teacher or sage who must be patient with the clearly stumbling steps of another, when in truth the other may simply have been behaving annoyingly, selfishly, cruelly, abusively, or perhaps out of fears of their own. Regardless, I had been unable to recognize that I don't have to allow myself to be subjected to certain situations, and that I am not responsible for the other's behavior.

Often in my witnessing process, echoes of former experiences appeared as familiar ripples within present circumstances, resounding deeply with the remembrance of a prior experience; new experiences showed up to pull out old responses so they could be acknowledged and released. As the feelings and memories came sliding out of hiding, I became more able to name the lie: the undivided truth of direct somatic re- experiencing cancelled out my inclinations to tell myself a different story about the initial experience or about the associated cascade of habitual patterns I had created to deflect this truth from my awareness. Almost always, there was pain. Always, there was sorrow. Then there was healing, as the locked energy of a long frozen state was released.

I began to feel empowered by irrefutable new insight regarding the futility of continuing as a 'noble martyr' through life; the inherent hypocrisy of such a state of being began to become clear to me. I had reached a 'catch 22' in which logic obliged me to acknowledge the previous habit of deflection and admit to myself that it was I who had been hurt by another; I had to absorb that the other one had, in fact, behaved inappropriately toward me. I began to see how my tendency to shift blame to myself was actually an attempt to regain control in face of feeling overwhelmed by circumstances external to myself.

This unfolding process began to reveal recurring themes, underneath which I found fear. I found myself asking: how deep is this well? What remains? Will it be empty? What fills the space that has been vacated and is now opening? Will wisdom find room to take root and expand?

The pattern of self-sabotage became evident again and again, as I slid down the vortex into inevitable feelings of despair and landed hard on the cold floor of primal awareness, where vigilance must prevail and higher aspirations must withdraw quietly into the corners. There, gradually, gently, came a dawning awareness of my deficit— my huge, insurmountable, never ending debt. What was this about? I came to see that I have been trying to pay for something I cannot pay for, a debt I can never pay, a debt that is not mine to pay and was never mine to pay. I have been feeling obliged to pay for the very right to my existence, the right for my essence to continue to exist.

Yet, my inner witness kept prompting me to dig deeper, telling me there is more to see and more to understand, that this point of view was not final. I had been duped, cajoled, lied to, and deceived into believing this thing about my very self that might not actually be true even though my very bones believed it was.

Why must I repeatedly push myself to a brink where I feel I have no choices, in order to allow myself permission to actually do what I must do? It's like a game I play with myself that I don't know how to win.

A word came, and came again—grace—and a silent instruction: *allow grace.* I saw grace on the bridge across the gulf between reality and potential, though I assumed it was not for me to cross it (because of, you know, *my deficit*). Yet, something within me knows beyond knowing that I am already on the way. When does perceived reality change from experiencing oneself as standing on the brink of this chasm to walking on the opposite side? How does one know the difference? Is *faith* a noun, a verb, or simply a concept we entertain intellectually as we gradually slide into a bubble of self-delusion, believing we are experiencing a phenomenon which is in fact an illusion? At which point does one cross over from imagining one is safe to knowing one is safe? How will I recognize the miracle unfolding while terror welcomes each in-breath and agony follows each breath back out? Will there ever be a time when it feels safe to simply breathe? What does it actually mean, to not feel safe?

My exploration into this frightening territory began to reveal its many meandering, interconnecting paths; broken bridges, endless loops, stagnant pools; dark tunnels and sheltering caves. Off in the distance of my deepest depths a voice was still screaming—this time, I resolved to follow it to its source. Through fold upon fold of half-told stories, echoing still amid shards of broken dream fragments, I persevered.

Gazing within, through the lens of current circumstance and my newfound understanding, I began to discern the undercurrent: the fact that I have been mired in concerns for survival finally began to surface. I have been stuck in the survival of my chosen life-style, my freedom to move about in life as I desire, and my ability to maintain myself effectively in this world, to pursue learning as I choose, to relate well with like-minded people, and to offer my gifts.

I also noticed a connection with unresolved issues of the chakras related to the more primal concerns of living. This showed itself as a deep inner conflict regarding beliefs related to my right to be here, relations with others, self-expression, thought processes, and so forth. This ambivalence was reflected in imbalances in my physical, emotional, mental, and behavioral states.

For example, in the root/self-preservation chakra, I had a pattern of striving with all my might to resolve my fears about being able to support myself effectively, yet persistently sabotaging my efforts through the cyclical manifestation of setbacks and roadblocks. I had been forced repeatedly to go back and start again from the point where I failed.

In the second chakra/creative centre, the urge to create beauty has repeatedly been contradicted by engagement in unhealthy relationships, sabotage of my artistically creative endeavors, and the persistence of addictive behaviors. My body has at various times reflected the inner conflict by producing hormonal and digestive imbalances resulting in distressing physical ailments.

As I began to become more aware of my energy field, I learned there was a deep tear in my third chakra. In my heart chakra, the imbalance showed in an ability to serve others with great compassion and yet an inability to allow myself to fully receive love. In the fifth chakra, self-restriction of my inner voice as well as suppression of my natural creative expression became evident. At the sixth, I became aware of habitually blinding my inner eye, refusing to allow myself to see what I see (what my perceptive abilities are showing me to be true).

At the crown chakra, perhaps my inner rebellion served me in a positive way. At an unusually young age I began to question the truth of what the 'authorities' were telling me in regard to reality, the Divine, and the nature of self and others. At this level I was able to recognize distortions and distinguish between wisdom and what was not necessarily the truth. This ability filtered through to my logic, where I felt no confusion about the contrast I saw between the fantasy presented to me as fact and my certainty that it was incorrect.

I began to suspect that my parents were, in fact, trying in the best way they knew how to protect me from things that had frightened and hurt them in their own lives, while at the same time feeling obligated to integrate their children into a community they were unfamiliar with.

Many years later as I reflect I am able to better understand the distortions and unhealed fears my parents themselves must have been struggling with in their own secret psyches. As I recognize my need to heal old wounds, to uncover unconscious beliefs, and to transform my inner reality, I often reflect upon my experience as a fifteen-year-old and try to see a little more clearly through the window this opened in my comprehension of causes and effects. From that time forward, it slowly began to dawn on me that adults were people, in the same way I was a person—someone who gets hurt, questions other peoples' views of reality, and wonders whether they are doing things correctly. I felt somehow less alone knowing that everyone else is also alone, at some deep level.

Now, in my mid-fifties, as I've followed the vibrating cords deep into my subconscious and made progress in resolving old issues, signs of something 'larger than my current life' also began to emerge. This 'something' seemed strangely familiar and felt very much like questions I had been asking in my childhood. "What is the universe? How far does it extend? It must end somewhere, but then, what exists beyond that"? Then came questions I asked as

I began transforming into a woman: "Who am I? Who am I to be? Where am I? Why am I here? What is the meaning of all this? What am I here to offer to the world?" Soon this evolved into "Do I exist beyond this physical existence? Will I still exist once I pass away from here? Am I safe? What is my role in the evolution of the universe? Will I be able to do my part well?

I came to see that my practice must be focussed on expanding my capacity to feel safe in an expanded environment, on understanding that choices are mine to make. My energy has been so focussed on survival that I haven't been in a position to fully direct my creativity to those elements I have been intending to develop.

Certain keynotes have been rising into the light of my conscious awareness, repeating again and again as an invitation. For example, I have begun to recognize my fear of remaining present, as well as my fear of entanglement, and have inquired more deeply into what this fear is about. I have found it is about not feeling safe when I am receptive and open unless I am alone in nature; deeply engaged in a creative project, learning something that truly interests me and stimulates both my mind and emotion; or serving another. When I am not engaged in this type of directed focus but am simply 'wide open', especially around other people, I have noticed a tendency to become agitated, anxious, and prone to deflecting the present moment. I had developed a habitual response of trying to escape from my body, while still engaging in the world through my body. I would somehow remain present enough to go through the motions while my imagination floated elsewhere. I struggled often with severe brain fog, not recognizing that I had dissociated—either as a result of boredom with having to learn something I saw no use for or as the result of anxiety related to a situation or association.

I am now beginning to understand the vulnerability I must have been feeling all my life as a highly sensitive, empathic individual. These new insights are enabling me to inquire more deeply into my own true nature without judging myself for my habitual responses to this anxiety. It is becoming quite liberating to be able to look for gifts in something that has seemed like such a frightful circumstance—and one for which I blamed myself. Another aspect arising repeatedly is the awareness of my discomfort with being one-with-myself, undivided. I can now see that a typical response has been to hide things from myself, to veil what I know to be true, to deny reality as it presents itself by going into fantasy mode—in effect, to fall into one of the various grooves making up the mask I have been using to shield myself from myself. I eventually came to the truth that I have not been completely honest with myself.

My work with somatic trauma release helped me begin to open a door I did not know was closed. Once it was drawn to my attention that one can only fully engage in life integrally through the body while on this earth, I was able to grasp the fuller meaning of what is meant by being present as an integrated whole being which includes the body, mind, and spirit. Why this should have come as a revelation is baffling to me, yet it has represented a turning point.

I came to understand that in order for healing to occur, it is necessary to stop apologizing for trying to describe or actually feel my own inner experience, regardless of how the circumstances may have looked from the outside. It is necessary to process and release the feeling that in admitting the devastating effects I personally experienced, I am betraying the other—whether this occurred at the hands of well-meaning (though frightened or misguided) adults who had no concept of the consequences of their behaviors, or arose in relationships I chose to engage in. Regardless of how it may sound, the important thing is a willingness to be honest with myself, to tell myself the truth. From here, I can begin to reconnect with the experience of my own body.

As I became more able to put self-judgement aside, I

began making rapid progress in my ability to revisit my past with greater objectivity and gain deeper understanding of the mechanisms holding my 'secret turmoil' in its frozen state. For example, in what I've referred to as 'fantasy mode'—a step beyond daydream, different from the floaty, dreamy state of my childhood—I've noticed a tendency to color reality, creating distortions in my sense of time lines and current capacities, in an attempt to come into the 'eye of the storm' and reinterpret a reality I perceive so painfully to exist. I began witnessing my brain-fogged state when it arises, my forward-curved shoulders as I anticipate further trauma, my shallow breathing as I engage in mental analysis or strategy, the rush of adrenalin as I react to being triggered, the pronounced tensing of muscles associated with anxiety. I have begun to recognize my tendency toward inner collapse by witnessing my body's tendency toward physical contraction, as well as my body relaxing as I open within. I am now learning that in listening to my body, I can more clearly decipher not only my emotional responses but also the messages coming through my higher perceptive faculties. Perhaps most importantly, I have become more able to recognize, and therefore to begin to unravel, my habitual response loops and their sources. It has become evident through this emotional/somatic level of experiencing that the loops often repeat at the same or greater intensity as to the original shock, even though the present event creating its recurrence may be far less severe in outward appearance.

Recently, I became aware of the sense of a ceiling or lid over the top of my head, and this sense has been making itself felt at various times throughout my days. As it comes to my attention, I reflect on the thoughts and emotions I had been entertaining and experiencing just prior. In regard to thoughts, the prevalent theme appears to be one of perceived limitations related to my ability to proceed along the path of my intention. A secondary theme has to do with fears that I will not be able to navigate in the world of interrelatedness with others as I shed my habitual self-protections. I began noticing that what arose emotionally had to do with feeling controlled, with a corresponding frustration magnifying into rage bubbling forth. Perhaps before my birth and then during my formative years, the ceiling was placed over me, and I am still—or have been—in that box of ancestral inheritance I must unravel and transcend. I have been rebelling against that box throughout my life, ironically, attracting more of it as I push against it with all my might.

A particularly prevalent aspect of ancestral inheritance that impacted me greatly had to do with the roles 'permitted' a woman. As I myself began to become a woman, I gradually recognized the 'lesser status' ascribed to females, not only within my inherited cultural group but also within the church community and society as a whole. The inner rebellion that arose within could not be allowed to emerge as overt, righteous anger or disobedience, as I perceived it unsafe to do so. I decided I must insist on equal personhood in more subtle ways. Besides this, I also began to notice such multigenerational themes as 'the need to work very hard in order to survive', 'luxuries are too extravagant to justify', 'children must obey and not question', 'correction is achieved through punishment', and so forth. I am certain there are many more to be discovered, intertwined in deep, subtle, and hidden ways with the threads of my beliefs.

The emotional cascade of repeated negative vortices began to serve as my cue to access the inner resources/inner discipline I have gradually been developing. By grounding, centering, and aligning while focussing consciously on deepening my breathing, I become more able to connect with my intention to expand my capacity for maintaining this alignment. The key discipline in this process is to refrain from collapsing inward, and from the subsequent impulse to flee (whether physically or mentally) that has been my habitual response to hurtful experiences as well as pleasant experiences that are outside my comfort zone. Once I succeed in staying present, I focus on consciously taking responsibility for having attracted my present circumstance, and for choosing to change my circumstance or to simply respond.

Recently I left work very anxious and upset. I walked as fast as I could and tears welled up, releasing some of the static from my nervous system. I practiced some grounding, centering, and aligning, with my hand on my solar plexus. I began to experience a felt sensation of being allowed now to let this trauma pattern heal—an inner knowing flooded through my body as I absorbed the warmth from my hand. I allowed myself some more time to become quiet inside, consciously feeling the strength of my legs carrying me, and then went back in to work, managing much better.

Once at home, I became aware of an emerging insight about how I've been unable to fully take advantage of the help offered me. This realization gave way to a deeper understanding about my inability to fully receive. As the evening progressed, and into the following day, I continued to have deeper and deeper insight into the entire pattern, right to its point of origin in my experience as a fifteen-year-old.

Further insights continued to occur spontaneously throughout the evening and next day. I recognized the building up of inner pressure echoed in my father's potential for volatility, and remembered suddenly how it felt to have to maneuver around this. In turn, I was able to understand how this tendency within him had in fact been part of a trauma he himself must have been experiencing. This led me to deeper insight regarding the events as I had walked into through the door that night. I suddenly understood that his behavior was rooted in some form of intense fear, that something he had perhaps heard or been told may have initiated a fear so intense, most likely for my safety, that it activated trauma within him. This must have led him to jump to an irrational conclusion, which in turn prompted his verbally violent behavior.

Once I recognized the fact that he must have experienced unbearable terror at some point(s) in his life in order to have such powerful reactions still active within his own nervous system, I began to feel a huge upwelling of compassion and sorrow for him, which led to further release of my own closed loop of locked energy. From there I became able to begin to renegotiate the pattern arising out of the original trauma, allow feelings of forgiveness to flow into my consciousness, and strengthen my capacity to experience compassion for myself.

Allowing myself to witness the cascading pattern and experience the somatic sensations released some of the locked energy, enabling me to absorb the healing sensations. I was now able to review the events of that night from a wider perspective. I started having more insight into why this event affected me so dramatically. I recalled how, at the campfire, alcohol and hash had been offered to me by others partaking in these substances. It was the first experience I'd had like that, and following my good sense, I refused. I felt good about having made a mature decision, and left it at that.

In the present, as I acknowledged my ability even as a fifteen-year-old to make good decisions, I began breathing more deeply, my shoulders relaxed, and my hips unclenched. What my parents could not have known is that, having done a very good job of alerting me to the potential for danger in the world, I had chosen wisely and assumed they would be proud, had they known about it. The irony of what took place instead, stripping me of all my psychological defenses, confounded the natural evolution of learning to trust in my own judgement.

Although I am not able to go back to that time and change anything, I am able now, in the present, to acknowledge something positive about myself. I am able to say, 'I was confronted with a challenge and met it well', and I can now allow myself to know that even back then, I was capable of making good choices. Perhaps more importantly, I can allow myself to feel good about this in the present and release self-blame for my father's behavior toward me.

Once I processed the trauma pattern and found a healing response, the memory of a similar and earlier, though less severe, event arose spontaneously. I had innocently offended my father and he had exploded into a tirade. I remember experiencing the familiar wash of chemicals inside my body as I tried to absorb the sudden, seemingly unprovoked scolding I was receiving. Only three years old at the time, I felt more stunned than traumatized, but perhaps that was enough to form a seed of doubt around which future experiences would begin swirling.

I recognize now the inner turmoil of an adult whose trauma had been triggered. I suddenly knew, inside myself, that I was not at fault for my father's unpredictable behaviors toward me—something in my body relaxed.

As I am learning to look for and recognize the solution within the problem, I am noticing that my perspective expands as I remove judgement from the equation. Catching myself when I engage in endless loops of self-criticism, consciously expanding my inner light while remaining centered from within my body, and thereby increasing the 'space' I occupy and can breathe within—all of this is enabling me to break open these habitual loops that all too easily begin spiralling down in a negative vortex. As I catch myself in the act, I begin to open space and allow a positive spiral to form and gain momentum. As I become more aware of the ways and extent to which I have been restricting myself, I am beginning to comprehend the difference between intending and then trying to control outcomes, and intending and allowing things to unfold. In turn, this is leading me to come again and again to insights regarding the mechanics of my role in having created that which I am engaged in, whether in struggle or joyously.

I begin to focus on compassion and healing for myself, which can only begin once I have remembered to give myself permission by acknowledging my right to be, here, now. I move my consciousness to my heart-space and allow myself to feel present reality from here. I can then move my attention to expanding the light from within, rippling outward and expanding my aura. In allowing the waves of old, ingrained patterns to rise to the surface for witnessing, I am able to clear trapped energy from my system. From this perspective, my mental process can move through the thoughts "I can do this" to "I will do this" to "I am doing this."

As I do these practices, I find I have arrived in a position from which I am able to shift my perspective to take in a broader view and see present circumstances within a larger context. This new seeing allows me to create space to recognize and follow the thread of hurt back to the event/experience that was the initial shock/wound. I clearly see how the series of effects rippling out from that point have formed a pattern through the time and space of my life, waiting only for the moment of my present awareness for resolution and healing. Depending on my degree of success at this moment of awareness, the pattern either begins to dissipate or arises again later in the form of a similar experience, so that I may try again to understand the lesson.

I'm beginning to recognize the state of tunnel vision I tend to slide into when I'm experiencing anxiety, and to become more adept at stepping back to view my circumstances as part of a bigger picture. From this new perspective I am able to discern more realistic options, rather than desperately jumping into potentially ineffective or even counterproductive 'solutions' just to get past this next part, and the next, and so on. This new skill is enabling me to begin to understand connections to earlier events and to renegotiate the trauma and its further reaching effects. As a result, I've been making some headway in restructuring circumstances that have been self-defeating, through simplification and ultimately greater efficiency in my approaches. This shift is only just beginning to be reflected in areas such as finances, interrelationship with others, and accepting my right to choose, though I still find myself stuck at the turning point between my previous career path and my present yearning to move in this new direction

Despite persistent life challenges, I'm becoming more able to distinguish between the feeling of fear about something and the actuality of its occurring—somehow I'd been experiencing them internally as the same thing. Very recently, as I was taking a walk I noticed a feeling of tension inside, which felt somehow different than the recently familiar tension associated with worry. I suddenly recognized it as a familiar feeling I've had in the past when working on a creative project. I identified it as creative tension I was experiencing in association with writing this paper. As I recognized the sensation from long ago, I suddenly remembered how I had firmly closed the door on art as I had begun to associate this form of positive tension with the tension of the stress I was feeling at that time. This awareness again produced a welling up of the pattern into my consciousness to be witnessed.

I'm becoming better able to distinguish what is and is not my responsibility, and to establish healthier boundaries. I'm learning about rhythm and momentum, giving myself permission to rest when I feel fatigued and to replenish myself. I'm learning to recognize my restrictive comfort zones and to expand into a healthier state of being, while also understanding that this, too, is a choice.

I'm finding that the more I practice using my inner resources as actual events occur, the more flexible I appear to be in using them adeptly, though it's a very gradual, unfolding process in the experiential realm. My progress feels slow as I continue to experience setbacks; yet as I become more able to witness the contracted state, I am becoming stronger as I once again expand, gradually replacing self-defeating patterns with self-nurturing routines. I remind myself that I am, in fact, embarked on a process of reinventing the wheel—the great wheel of my life—and understanding that my life is worthy of being whole, without apology or justification, simply because I am. I'm learning that forgiveness is an act of self-love, and that self-love is necessary for true healing.

An important aspect of this process has been the allowance for mistakes, with related learning about forgiveness and gentleness toward myself, others, life, and the universe— even the Divine. I come to see mistakes in a different light, not as terrible black marks on the soul for which I deserve to be punished and eternally condemned, but as the natural steps in a learning process. When I amplify this concept to the greater scale and regard mistakes as the natural steps in the learning process of the soul as it evolves and unfolds toward the Light of its own magnificence, my sense of context opens until I feel inspired by my growing understanding that THIS IS REALITY; I AM PART OF THIS MAGNIFICENT REALITY.

Arriving

I arrive, finally, at the realization that I am not only permitted self-healing, but that this is the only place I can really begin from if I would heal and transform myself, the world, and all of creation. Paradoxically, while making the assumption that it is arrogant to aspire to engage in such a lofty role, I had inadvertently become arrogant by setting myself apart from All That Is, thinking myself unworthy to be that which I truly am. With this realization, I find myself feeling truly humble for the first time. As I expand my ability to be still inside and to stay quiet, I notice myself listening. I settle, finally, into my heart space, and find myself beginning to receive inner guidance of a higher order than my mind is able to supply. I recognize the voice which has been whispering to me all through my life, though I struggled to stop my ears by inventing many dimensions of experience I now must admit were distortions of truth.

As I begin to recognize myself as a whole being once more—a consciously transforming whole being—I find myself remembering the natural wisdom of my childhood. As I step forth knowing myself now as an adult, I may put aside the things of childhood while allowing the memory of this earlier wisdom to teach me. It is a thing I have consciously been striving to do for many years, at times believing I was whole enough and becoming successful. Yet had I achieved the ability to hold myself in a state of inner stillness amidst external circumstances, witnessing and participating in the events of life while centered within? Had I managed to step forth, not disconnected from life, but rather moving through experiences with the dignity of inner poise? Had I arrived at a point of balance characterized not by disassociation from external circumstances, but rather by viewing them through the compassion of the heart, from the wisdom that comes with the understanding that true compassion must also encompass self? I could argue that I have been striving to do these things for a long time, yet I was truly unable to encompass my own self in the compassion of my heart until now.

The *experiential* understanding that I must allow healing for myself in order to be of true service to others may be the underlying learning on this journey of arriving at a sense of being safe, a certain knowing that my attentive focus can shift from one of primary survival concerns to creative participation in life. It is the shift from understanding this concept mentally to embodying this understanding experientially that is propelling me forward. Finally having become able to acknowledge I was not feeling safe in my life, in the world, or in the universe, I am coming nearer now to stepping into a place where I not only know I am always safe, but am able to live from this place.

Evolution is a process, not only of continuous adaptation, but also of creativity in motion. What is this creative force propelling life forward in this way? How can individuals possibly be 'apart' from this Flow of Intelligent Energy, this Divine Breath of Consciousness becoming manifest? How can I possibly be apart from the Great Mystery, whatever its true nature? I cannot be separate from this, and therefore, as I continue along on my journey home, I may yet come to know myself as I AM, and as a part of THAT I AM.

This is Julia's story—a profound reflection of where she is today. Sri Aurobindo names the process:

> There is a stage in the sadhana in which the inner being begins to awake. Often the first result is the condition made up of the following elements: 1. A sort of witness attitude in which the inner consciousness looks at all that happens as a spectator or observer... 2. A state of neutral equanimity...in which there is quietude... 3. A sense of being something separate from all that is happening, observing it but not part of it. 4. An absence of attachment to things, people or events [with]...an inner peace and silence...a positive sense of calm...there should be no going out of the body...there should be a perfect awareness of all that is going on in or around you...if you can concentrate in the heart as well as in the head, then these things can more easily come. (Ghose, 1995, pp. 1002-1003).

We now turn to Part Three and examine human becoming, Gnostic transformation, and the path of return process within the context of Integral yoga developed here. We also address notions of rebirth and karma, and close with ideas related to lighting the flame of inquiry, taking Part Two and Julia's story into consideration.

PART THREE:
HUMAN BECOMING

14
THE PATH OF RETURN:
FROM SADHANA TO PSYCHE

In this chapter we examine human becoming and provide a synthesis of what we have discussed while adding more complexity in terms of the soul and psychic being—the living sacred heart aspect of Integral yoga. Following this, we examine rebirth and karma, and address the processes that support yogic individuation from within the context of Integral yoga developed here. We close with ideas related to where we have been in terms of this perspective of Integral yoga as the original research informed it and this extension of the research develops it, and examine how ongoing and future work can advance soul- centered living. The epilogue provides a preliminary reflection on how the emotional-vital aspect of Integral yoga could be— indeed, may be—reflected in global, community, and individual living-in-the-world today.

As we have seen, the human personality is multilevel and capable of expressing itself in many ways. However, according to Integral yoga, one single consciousness underlies all we do and all we are: this consciousness can be called Brahman, and is given other names in different spiritual traditions. From the surface consciousness and its many aspects, turning inward, leading through deeper and deeper levels of consciousness to the *Brahman consciousness*, the path is fraught with challenges to this surface egoic consciousness. How does one journey inward? What is involved? Where does one start?

Sri Aurobindo (Ghose, 2000a) outlines three methods by which to activate the evolutionary changes—methods that open the way to a consciousness he terms Brahman consciousness, which is one gained by the true mystics and yogis. However, for our purposes Sri Aurobindo's method articulates a developmental process that leads individuals away from the explicate, materialistic, matter-bound, unhealthy egoic, relative, and often meaningless orientation exclusive to the external, toward an alignment with an inner centre sometimes called the ground of being.

Of the three main methods, Sri Aurobindo recommends the route through the psychic or soul as the safest and least likely to trigger egoic power states or trap individuals in an occult state of astral illusion. A second method focuses above the head, accessing the higher states of mind and supermind consciousness. However, this opening to higher consciousness can lead to a split between the personality and the higher self as individuals are tempted to remain in a bliss-based higher consciousness and may become averse to integrating the two— perhaps in denial of lower behaviors. The third method focuses at the ajna point between the eyes, which can be very powerful once activated; however, Sri Aurobindo cautions that there remains a real danger individuals using this method may become caught in a state of magnified ego, adrift in cosmic illusion and Ignorance (Ghose, 1996, 2000c).

The safest and surest route, activation of the soul, begins with a process that opens the inner-heart so that soul energies can come forward. To Sri Aurobindo (Ghose, 2000a), the soul is the innermost part of our being: the true master directing our life. He says that the soul is a Divine "nucleus pregnant with possibilities" projected into Matter to bring forth an awakening so Matter can return to the Divine (p. 288). Hence, inner spiritual movement is present, consciously or unconsciously, and acts as a 'secret witness' to all we say and do. While present in our lives, the soul can be shrouded by ignorance or egoic tendencies, yet it remains ever aware of the call to evolve— unless, as Sri Aurobindo states, it has retreated in despair, perhaps to return at another time or in another lifetime. Sri Aurobindo believes that most people are unaware of their soul, and of the psychic being that develops as a form and expression of it.

The psychic being is an aspect of the soul, itself unborn and surviving life and death; it manifests in each lifetime, standing behind the surface personality. Sri Aurobindo (Ghose, 2000a, 2000b) describes the psychic being as a spark of the Divine formed by the soul, and soul growth as bringing forth experiences into our lives that enhance the evolution of the soul. The psychic being is the soul of the person evolving in manifestation, growing each time the individual makes a higher choice; at first veiled, often dominated by the lower personality forces, it nevertheless provides guidance through indirect influence. The psychic being comes forward over lifetimes through a process called sadhana. It is, however, an actual being with a subtle form or a conscious individuality, also known as the central being because it is the force that directs our lives in the process toward self-realisation. As the Mother says, the psychic being is the secret cause that turns us God-ward and provides unerring guidance, birthing a psychic individuality far greater than the egoic individuality of the outer personality (Ghose, 2000a; Dalal, 2002). It is the soul in the secret heart focusing us (either covertly or overtly) toward right feeling, right thought, right perception, and right attitude.

The Mother says that when an individual is near death,

> the psychic being is still in the body and has noted what it has learnt, it decides for the next occasion. And sometimes it is a movement of action and reaction: because it has studied one entire field, it needs to study the opposite field. And very often if chooses a very different life from one it had. (Ghose, 1999, p. 74).

She adds, "before if comes down, it looks for the kind of vibration it wants; it sees them very clearly" (p. 75) and in response, there must be receptivity or aspiration from below, usually a "small light" kindled from the new mother.

Still, she continues, in most people the psychic being remains unconscious. "In ordinary life there is not one person in a million who has conscious contact with his psychic being, even momentarily" (Ghose, 1999, p. 48)—it is left to work quietly from within. Conversely, there are exceptions "where the psychic being is an entirely formed, liberated being, or master of itself, which has chosen to return to earth in a human body in order to do its work" (p. 48). It becomes a "worker upon earth to help in the fulfillment of the Divine work" and progresses through that work (p. 64).

For most of us the Mother recommends making the mind silent and then entering deeply into the heart, beyond all sensation. She notes that, at first, contact with the psychic being is sporadic but continued effort produces results—a great joy comes forth and an extreme sweetness accompanies this interiorized state (Ghose, 1999).

Together the soul and its representative psychic being are accessed through the heart: the inner heart that rests behind the desire-heart or emotional-heart (Dalal, 2005). Dalal describes how contact with the soul usually develops through sadhana, a turning-inward process often initiated by shock, grief, and other serious disruptions to the egoic way of being. Sadhana is defined here as a yogic process that serves to push the individual inward, creating a tension—sometimes a very painful tension—that serves to open pathways to the inner heart (Ghose, 2000a).

Sadhana elicits a slow wisdom-building that creates openings to the inner heart, openings to higher order vibrations, a broader spectrum of knowledge, and a loosening of the narrow egoic-ideation states. The result is an increasing sense of freedom, caring, joy, and a clarity more sensitive to, as Sri Aurobindo says, the "true and good and beautiful, fine and pure and noble" (Dalal, 2005, p. xx). As the egoic encrustations crack, allowing more energetic connectivity of flow between the inner and outer worlds, there is an "upbuilding of divinity in the earthy nature" says Dalal (p. xxxi) that results in the transformative growth of the soul. There is a freedom from the "bondage and suffering imposed by life, mind and body" (p. xxxi).

Why is suffering imposed, and how do life, mind, and body impose this suffering? To some degree, suffering seems to be integral to the human condition and is cited as a state to be overcome by the world's great spiritual traditions.

In Integral yoga, as we discussed earlier, Sri Aurobindo (Ghose, 1996) outlines a profoundly hopeful and helpful explanation based on the notion of involution and evolution. Specifically, Matter is consciousness involved to the state of Inconscience; in other words, consciousness is so involved that it is unaware of its consciousness. Evolution is growing consciousness, awakening consciousness, the bringing forth of the involved consciousness from Matter through the stages of mineral, plant, animal, and human. For the human, the unfolding of consciousness is a process fraught with challenges, as the inertia of the inconscience and the coarseness of Ignorance gives way to an ever evolving awareness.

This ever evolving awareness is itself steeped in complexity: Sri Aurobindo (Ghose, 1996) speaks of a process that reaches from inconscience, to ignorance, to a culmination in an ever-evolving supramental consciousness. However, within the context of transformation, it is the outward physical, emotional- vital, and mental consciousness that contribute to the raw material of the egoic, fixed patterning within each of us. Soul energy can then use the stress created to promote an opening for this very habit-bound, patterned vehicle of physical, vital, and mental to humbly (often nonconsciously) connect to the waiting soul energies; these energies bring forth lessons and insights, and open the pathway to the inner, wiser, subtle physical, vital, and mental processes. Julia's story elucidates this process masterfully (see Chapter 13).

While it may not take suffering to awaken the opening to soul, it often does take at least a time of dissonance and discomfort of sufficient force to loosen the hold of old ways of being. According to Sri Aurobindo, to awaken the soul—or rather, to awaken the outer being to the consciousness of the soul— requires a pressure from the psychic being, or a pressure from above, from the higher levels of mind above the intellect (Ghose, 2000a, 2000b). At some point, this pressure is felt by the outer planes of being—the physical, vital, or mental.

For the soul to inform the outward life, the physical, emotional-vital, and mental planes of being must be impacted; otherwise, individuals will remain caught in the illusory, surface, external world of matter and will view material life as an end in itself rather than as an expression of the soul in matter. These planes do not sense the originator, spirit, or self-aware consciousness—Atman (Ghose, 2000a). Both the subjective personality and these outer planes of being are but formations of this greater consciousness, and there are vast ranges of consciousness above and below this very finite, outer human formation.

As noted above, there are both inner and outer planes of physical, emotional-vital, and mental consciousness. The outer physical (meaning the gross physical) is the body, the outward senses, and the cellular structures as they inform and create the physical structure and function. There is also an inner subtle physical—an energy-body physical that is pliable, plastic, and interpenetrates and extends beyond the physical body. The emotional-vital (also referred to as the life-force in the outer nature) can be an awkward force of Ignorance ruling the outer being, and can be taken over by hostile forces that then rule the outer being. Sri Aurobindo (Ghose, 1996) says that the inner emotional-vital is more receptive to the rule of the soul and the higher mind, and it can then become a powerful servant of spiritual development. Finally, the outer or lower mental being guides via egoic thought, and is based on external world patterns, habits, and cultural norms. The inner mental has access to the higher ideals, values, and guidance from the soul or from the higher mental planes. But, as we saw with Julia (Chapter 13), accessing these higher planes takes sustained effort—tapasya.

In the average person, the lower planes of being are separate from the inner, more conscious planes; the inner planes enhance awareness and provide actions with the substance of truth and the force that makes it easier to choose the right thoughts, emotions, and actions. Sri Aurobindo (Ghose, 2000a) reminds us that as the veils of Ignorance become thinner, higher levels of consciousness— right to the supramental consciousness— can and do transform one's body, life, and mind. He clearly advises individuals to find ways to free themselves from the limitations of the ordinary physical, emotional-vital, and mental formations that hold them in separation from their inner, wise, sacred centre, from each other, and from Divine consciousness.

Sri Aurobindo (Ghose, 2000a, 2000b) outlines a complex outer structure of physical, emotional-vital, and mental planes of being located between the inner physical, emotional-vital, and mental on the one hand, and this innermost subliminal proper or psychic being on the other. Each of these between planes is a world of its own having forces, forms, and beings that, he says, exist for their own purposes. From an outer perspective, each plane appears indistinct yet it is possible to discern the types of consciousness inherent in each of these three planes of being. Access to these states comes with sadhana and requires a softening of the ego, an upward aspiration, and an opening to an involutionary descent of consciousness.

Remember, Sri Aurobindo (Ghose 2000a, 2000b) discusses the different subplanes within the outer physical, vital, and mental planes of the earth-consciousness. For example, the physical plane has a submental-based mental-physical characterized by habit, impulse, and instinct that is capable of resisting higher mental instructions, especially when illness is present. A vital-physical consciousness is also present on this plane, connected to the nervous system, as is a material- physical, cellular consciousness that is resistant to change but immensely important in providing life-force for the physiology and protection of the body. When the inner subtle physical is activated, more substantial guidance from the psychic being and the inner realms of the emotional-vital and mental can be directed through diligent effort; this effort can give the material-physical a more pliable, plastic harmony. The Mother spent many years attempting to bring the higher consciousness directly into the physical body at the cellular level (Pandit, 1992).

The emotional-vital plane is also multidimensional. The lower vital-physical, a level steeped in small desires, is closely connected to the nervous system via the lower physical-vital; hence the strong physical-emotional interconnections in health and illness. Highly driven by desire and emotion, this lower vital aspect automatically strives to fulfill its desires and immerse itself in emotion, whether anger, fear, jealousy, greed, or pleasure. With its seat in the navel, it seeks to enhance the sensations associated with egoic consciousness through the power and force of the smaller will. The higher emotional-vital in the heart centre is nearer the vital-emotional-mind, and more open to the influence of the mind and the deeper call of the heart; the higher emotional-vital provides a mental expression for the feelings and emotions stirred in the vital being and interprets higher insights, intuitions, and imagination.

Openings to the higher vital are instrumental for spiritual growth, and this transformation is powered by an inwardly directed life-force; however, the assistance of the planes of mind and the psychic being is required to overcome the vital plane's strong propensity for illusion, suffering, and perverse, seeming delight in the lower desire nature. When this happens, the true emotional-vital and the inner being higher vital advocate for the soul's life—growth of the psychic being occurs with amazing courage and a wide, calm strength.

Addressing the cognitive aspects of our being with intelligence, ideas, thoughts, and perceptions, the plane of mind also has dimensional aspects. The physical-mind is the mind of the cells and molecules, structured in its function and resistant to change. The physical-mind is concerned with sense data alone—the visible, tangible, and material. The vital-mind, or emotional-vital mind is the imaginative mind and the creative, dreaming mind; it sets up ideas for the future and tries to enact them. This can activate the thought-mind to focus on ideas, thought-forms, concepts, and theories. Sri Aurobindo says that the thought-mind is often a servant of the vital mind; however when the spiritual-mind is directed inward, accessing the psychic being or being accessed by the psychic being, it becomes steeped in Truth, aware of the Self, and open to receive higher knowledge (Ghose, 2000b).

In summary, the outer complex planes of being hold us captive until—either through developmental advancement or the grace of the psychic being's influence—we turn inward. With this turn, we activate the subtle physical, the inner vital, and the inner mental, so that the subliminal proper or psychic being can come forth to direct and guide our life and spiritual advancement. Sri Aurobindo provides hope as he reiterates:

> And while on the surface we are cut off from all around us except through an exterior mind and sense-contact which delivers but little of us to our world or of our world to us, in theses inner reaches the barrier between us and the rest of existence is thin and easily broken; there we can feel at once—not merely infer from their results, but feel directly—the action of the secret world-forces, mind- forces,

life-forces, subtle physical forces that constitute universal and individual existence.... (Ghose, 1996, p.171).

The inner planes become our guide. However, below the outer plane and deep within the inner planes of physical, emotional- vital, and mental lies a formidable foe that is also a formidable ally in ensuring our sadhana continues: the realm of the subconscious.

Not only do the planes of being play an immensely important role in the evolution of consciousness, Sri Aurobindo adds a whole new dimension of complexity to the healing process when he addresses the subconscient.

This frontal and external being is a confused amalgam of mind-formations, life-movements, physical functioning of which even an exhaustive analysis into its component parts and machinery fails to reveal the whole secret. It is only when we go behind, below, above into the hidden stretches of our being that we can know it: the most thorough and acute surface scrutiny and manipulation cannot give us the true understanding or the completely effective control of our life, its purposes, its activities; that inability indeed is the cause of the failure of reason, morality and every other surface action to control and deliver and perfect the life of the human race. For below even our most obscure physical consciousness is a subconscious being in which as in a covering and supporting soil are all manner of hidden seeds that sprout up, unaccountably to us, on our surface and into which we are constantly throwing fresh seeds that prolong our past and will influence our future, - a subconscious being, obscure, small in its motions capriciously and almost fantastically subrational, but of immense potency for the earth-life. (Ghose, 1996, pp. 170-171).

The subconscient is a repository for all that the conscious outer mind has repressed either consciously or unconsciously—it remembers all and can carry forth information from previous lifetimes. Out of habit it will repeatedly throw forth ideas, thoughts, images, or emotions to be captured by the dream state or the lower physical, emotional-vital, or mental. Sri Aurobindo (Ghose, 1996) believes that the subconscient provides a formidable resistance to any attempted change of consciousness. It seeks status quo in inertia, obscurity, and weakness, propelling outward its small fears, anxieties, and desires. Being aware of the necessity for transformation here is crucial; nevertheless, Sri Aurobindo cautions, the route to change in the subconscient is to utilize the psychic being and to focus on the positive nature of purification. These actions, when primary, allow one to (secondarily) clearly direct the subconscient via the forces of right attitude and right consciousness on both the outer and inner planes of being. Over time this direction imprints the subconscient, shifting the detractor-consciousness to supportive-consciousness.

While Sri Aurobindo (Ghose, 2000b) highlights a number of avenues that can successfully provide the opening to higher ways of being, we focus here on the pathway of the heart and the journey to deepening the connection with the psychic—the soul. In this journey, the concept of the subliminal is an important aspect. The subliminal consciousness is an amazing connector consciousness, larger than the surface waking consciousness, potentially luminous, filled with higher wisdom, fluid, and more open to the truth from a higher divine source. This unique, subtle, and expanded consciousness provides a larger, freer, efficient mind that lies behind the outer mind—a larger, more powerful, more subtle, divine emotional-vital behind the outer vital; and a subtler, more plastic, more fluid physical behind the gross physical. For most of us, it rests behind a veil while holding access to the true eternal self, the soul, the unborn Spirit, Brahman, and ironically, to the lesser yet powerful ways of being (Ghose, 1996, 2000a, 2000b).

Sri Aurobindo discusses the subliminal in a number of ways in his works. He refers to it as all that is not conscious (i.e., all that is not in the aware consciousness) and as all that is circumconscient, including the environment. Sri Aurobindo also speaks of subliminal knowledge and subliminal Ignorance (Ghose, 1996). In another view, Sri Aurobindo refines his focus and differentiates the subliminal from all that is not in the unconscious, not in the subconscious, while more clearly defining the subliminal as all that is in the higher consciousness (Dalal, 2005). Dalal states that Sri Aurobindo understands the waking mind and ego, and the outer physical, emotional-vital, and mental to be superimposed on a large, submerged, and subtle subliminal consciousness. Of note, Dalal claims that Sri Aurobindo identifies the innermost subliminal proper as the psychic being. Dalal also says that little is known about the subliminal in either Western or yogic philosophy.

In this context, the "inner mental, inner vital, inner more subtle physical reaches supported by an inmost psychic existence which is the connecting soul of all the rest" (Ghose, 1996, p. 171) specifically provide the safest bridge between the worlds such that integral consciousness can be embraced. Transformation requires the ability to push past the normal, ordinary, superficial waking-consciousness to access the vast concealed consciousness. Greater capacities of knowing and experiences are available in this "concealed self" (Dalal, 2005, p. 22). Through sadhana, the inner consciousness begins to open, until eventually the sadhak (seeker) lives more and more in the complex inner being. Dalal assures us that as individuals become more responsive to the psychic being, the subliminal opens upward to the unborn eternal spirit. However, Dalal also speaks of the subliminal as a "meeting place of consciousness that emerges from below by evolution" and descends from above by involution (p. 24).

The subliminal is not hampered by the superficial physical, emotional-vital, and mental because it has the capacity to be powerful and luminous and is the source of thoughts, feelings, motives, and actions—virtually all the personality's operative energies. However, powerful energy centres mediate the mundane-cosmic interconnection so that "only a little of the inner being escapes through these centres—the best part is mostly closed or asleep" (Dalal, 2005, p. 26). As these centres or chakras open, the powers and possibilities of the inner being and psychic being are aroused and in turn awaken the larger subliminal consciousness—and following this, the cosmic consciousness.

Sri Aurobindo (Ghose, 1999) speaks of integral methods for approaching and enhancing the clarity of soul and higher mind in order to overcome the lower triple world of physical, emotional-vital, and mind. The safest path for the ladder of transcendence, he assures us, is to focus on the psychic and utilize the force of the psychic being. He suggests bringing the power of concentration to the heart centre with the purpose of opening this centre through aspiration and loving surrender. And, he reminds us, resistance to this process is part of Universal Nature, as this Nature does not want individuals "to escape from the Ignorance into the Light" (p. 122). Resistance to the soul-ward movement may take the form of a vehement insistence on the continuation of the old movements, waves of them thrown on the mind and vital and body so that old ideas, impulses, desires, feelings, responses continue even after they are thrown out and rejected, and can return like an invading army from outside, until the whole nature given to the Divine, refuses to admit them (p. 122).

The challenge is great, as the internal is hidden by the powerful structure of the external consciousness:

> This materialized soul lives bound to the physical body and its narrow superficial external consciousness, and it takes normally the experiences of its physical

organs, its senses, its matter-bound life and mind, with at most some limited spiritual glimpses, as the whole truth of existence. (Ghose, 1996, p. 447)

The universal is veiled behind the individual way-of-being, all senses are turned to the external, consciousness is fractured, and the life that is lived is only a minute aspect of all that is available to humankind.

Sri Aurobindo (Ghose, 1996) speaks eloquently of Nature's 'hold' on this separated individual; in particular, he clearly outlines the power and force held within the emotional-vital or life-force consciousness. He describes how its power-play is dominated by desire, keeping us rajasically seeking external satisfaction. Should we remain external on the vital plane, we are seekers of experiences and possessions, fulfilling an unending array of needs. However, if one turns inward to the inner vital without initially activating the psychic being, the subliminal world is entered without the safety and wisdom provided by the soul. The individual then taps into a "life-world or desire-world hidden in us, a secret consciousness in which life and desire find their untrammeled play and their easy self-expression and from there throw their influences and formations in our outer life" (p. 449). Sri Aurobindo elaborates the risks of this state of awareness:

> In proportion as the power of this vital plane manifests itself in [an individual] and takes hold of [his or her] physical being, this [man or woman] of earth becomes a vehicle of the life energy..(p.449).

This person is soon out of control and rajasic energies create wild desires, uncontrollable desires, intense passions, and emotions that lead to actions—actions that can build and soon become out of control, destructive and dangerous to humanity.

According to Sri Aurobindo, the greater danger is that the darker forces from this inner plane can become attracted to individuals in this state and can magnify desire such that the individual becomes racked by a force of unlimited desire and passion and hunted and driven by an active capacity and colossal rajasic ego, but in possession of far greater and more various powers than those of the [individual] in the ordinary more inert earth-nature. (Ghose, 1996, p. 449).

> The desire-world will eventually pull this person down, creating an even greater separation from the soul. As with the emotional-vital, the mental opening to the inner is also fraught with complications when the soul force is not highly active. There is a subliminal unknown and unseen concealed behind this waking consciousness and visible organism this mental soul, mental nature, mental body and a mental plane, not materialized, in which the principle of Mind is at home and not as here at strife with a world which is alien to it, obstructions to its freedom and corruptive of its purity and clearness. (Ghose, 1996, p. 450).

When the transformation process opens, "all the higher faculties in man, his intellectual and psycho-mental being and powers, his higher emotional life awaken and increase in proportion as this mental plane in him presses upon him." (p. 451). Here the temptation is to leave the world—to become the recluse, the yogi in the cave. This person

> ...would enjoy powers and a vision and perceptions beyond the scope of ordinary life and body; he would govern all by the clarities of pure knowledge; he would be united to other beings by a sympathy of love and happiness; his emotions would be lifted to the perfection of the psychomental plane, his sensations rescued from grossness, his intellect subtle, pure and flexible, delivered from the deviations of the impure pranic energy and the obstructions of matter (p. 452).

Sri Aurobindo expresses the extreme of the yogi or mystic who become Self-realized through the mind leaving earth-plane work; such yogis become removed from the evolutionary process undertaken in the presence of life as it is lived while embracing the lower triple being.

The physical body also has a subtle physical, astral, multidimensional field surrounding the body that carries the subliminal consciousness information related to the internal workings of the body, information about the environment, and access to information at a distance. As we saw in Part Two, activating the subtle physical and astral comes with its own dangers if it is not done in conjunction with the activation of the psychic being.

In his writings, Sri Aurobindo (Ghose, 1999, 2000a, 2000b) patiently reminds us that the evolution of consciousness and the evolution of humankind will occur right here on the planet. It is a fierce journey fraught with complexities and dangers, as can be seen; nevertheless, he outlines methods to approach the inner planes.

Sadhana or yogic practice is a process of opening the consciousness to the psychic, to the Divine, ensuring that the passage from earth to heaven and back is guided by the wisdom of existence, consciousness, and bliss, or sachchidananda (Ghose, 1996). The psychic being, the Mother reminds us, is the secret cause behind all turning to the divine. As individuals respond, the psychic being becomes more progressively formed around the divine centre or soul. The more the psychic being guides, consciously or not, the more powerful the inner subliminal becomes in bringing down the universal force of cosmic life. Sri Aurobindo tells us the soul with its seat behind the heart provides not knowledge, "but an essential or spiritual feeling—it has the clearest sense of the Truth and a sort of inherent perception of it which is of the nature of soul- perception and soul-feeling" (Ghose, 1999, p. 17). He reminds us:

It is our inmost being and supports all the others, mental, vital, physical, but it is also much veiled by them and has to act upon them as an influence rather than by its sovereign right of direct action; its direct action becomes normal and preponderant only at a high stage of development or by yoga (p. 17).

Sadhana brings the psychic being forward, activating the soul attributes and thereby strengthening the bond with Truth as the inner planes are penetrated and new ways of being are determined. *Mukti* or liberation (or degrees of this state) comes with the slow process of sadhana. Sri Aurobindo (Ghose, 2000b) affirms the intricate processes of aspiration, rejection, and surrender, and in order to activate these traits he recommends the development of a witness consciousness—an awakened consciousness that brings with it the ability to step back. This sophisticated movement requires an awareness of the lower planes, that is, the physical, emotional-vital, and mental.

In terms of aspiration, the witness state is plastic, awake, aware, and able to discern when the power and force of the lower physical, emotional-vital, or mental is out of alignment with the psychic being—as Julia describes in chapter thirteen. In other words, silent nudges from the soul can interpenetrate through to the lower consciousness because the witness consciousness has been activated. The mind has become silent enough to 'hear', to provide a space for the descent of knowing that carries right attitude. The aspiration that has already been set within the consciousness opens the way for this process.

Rejection is the next stage, where the sadhak must be able to separate the ego from the soul consciousness or higher inner awareness. Masquerading as soul and often using the outer or inner vital resources, the ego will sabotage the movement of rejection. The physical-nature consciousness, bound by its inertia and engrained routines, also supports the life-force of the vital desire-nature. Sri

Aurobindo (Ghose, 2000b) cautions us that at this point—unless our aspiration is burning like a flame, completely vigilant—individuals will succumb to the false desires of the ego. That is why it is necessary to first develop a healthy-enough ego, then to see the Beyond ego. The mind, in stillness and receptive to the witness consciousness, must be kept open to the truth which thereby empowers the psychic being; without this quietude and equanimity, the vital nature's demands, cravings, and hostility to Truth will overcome the individual. Interestingly, Sri Aurobindo cautions against the folly of a weak vital as well, as a weak vital "shakes at every descent" (Pandit, 1992, p. 24) and cannot sustain the will to aspire for Truth. He reminds us that a strong physical body is also required, as the emotional-vital will weaken a body that cannot sustain its force for vital energy that both gives and draws.

Once the witness consciousness is working in conjunction with a clear and quiet mind such that soul guidance can be received, then surrender is the next step. This is a process of self-consecration. Individuals are asked to release all personal, lower egoistic ideas, feelings, and impulses, and utilize all the resources of the healthy ego to access guidance held by a higher freedom and a nobler perfection. Sri Aurobindo (Pandit, 1992) explains how this process of surrender replaces effort— something else in us, a higher, sweeter, truer force, guides our life. Of course, he cautions, this is not tamasic surrender but surrender that requires a new kind of effort grounded in dynamic, active, and courageous faith that can grow and sustain this process. Again, he cautions, this is not an egoistic faith designed to satisfy the lower nature, and not a "low smoke obscured flame that cannot burn upwards to heaven" (p. 30), but a pure flame that burns upward and inward, accessing the psychic sense of soul-knowing.

Sri Aurobindo discusses the unique traits of surrender: "consciousness, plasticity and unreserved surrender. For you must be conscious in your mind and soul and heart and life and the very cells of your body" (Pandit, 1992, p. 108). Individuals are to seek an "awakened and living communion" with the psychic being, and thereby with the divine presence, Brahman (p. 108). Conscious progress lends itself to plasticity in surrender because the awakened inner mind and inner vital directed toward the psychic being are sustainers of the divine force. In addition, Sri Aurobindo says, "even the body will awake and unite at last its consciousness to the supramental consciousness force" (p. 109). The foundation is reason and mind, but nevertheless faith, sustained by the psychic being, goes far beyond the realm of the "half-lit" lower mind (p. 110).

To gain self-awareness, which is a major component of transformation, Sri Aurobindo encourages individuals to open their souls to the Divine, allow the psychic being to sense truth consciousness, and develop inner perception. Persistence is necessary, with an understanding of the play of Natural law versus Divine Presence, for as he affirms, "there are many tangled knots that have to be loosened and cannot be cut abruptly asunder" (Pandit, 1992, p. 113). Knots, entanglements, or grooves created over time and lifetimes by the lower triple consciousness require a slow loosening so that integral consciousness can slowly and safely come forth through a grounded self-awareness— hence the need to work from within the nexus of 'readiness'.

Integral yoga—a comprehensive yoga—is designed to bring self-awareness, self-transcendence, and transformation. A path- of-return, it aims to heal the split between the lower and higher planes through the process of ascent and descent of consciousness utilizing the psychic being. Pandit (1983) states:

> When you move to the higher consciousness, to a higher level of being, you do not let the other levels drop; you come down, assimilate them and then go upwards ... at each step onward, upward and inward, he has to inject that consciousness in the other parts, impart character to the rest of his

existence and only when that is fairly organized, can he think of the next step. This is the meaning of 'all life is Yoga': integral scope and integration at every step (p. 72).

Sri Aurobindo and the Mother elucidate an ancient yogic path to transformation and teach a sophisticated and deeply caring approach. They do not ignore the ugly, fierce, or frightening, and instead speak the truth of a path fraught with challenges yet capable of leading to the highest realization: Brahman consciousness, a consciousness of Oneness. Moreover, they uniquely honor the yogic individuation associated with the earth-walk, pointing the way to a mystical and pragmatic marriage of heaven and earth.

In this marriage and on this path of return, Sri Aurobindo elucidates a perspective on karma and rebirth. His is a useful view for individuals seeking deeper and alternative views of the human condition.

INTEGRAL REFLECTIONS:

OLD ME—NEW ME
10 STEP INTEGRAL TRANSFORMATION PROCESS

1. Notice the issue or the problem: physical, emotional/ somatic, mental and/or spiritual.
   Note the signal or the dissonance.

2. Connect with the issue, then step back and again deeply connect with the issue.
   Step back and widen consciousness.

3. Deconstruct the story using Witness consciousness.
   Remember there are varieties of witness consciousness: sattwic, rajasic, tamasic.

4. Identify distorted patterns—that is, physical, emotional/ somatic, mental, and spiritual belief sets.
   Consider pattern recognition, meta-pattern, meta-meta- pattern. Think about your styles of thinking, such as thought-mind, uncover vital/ emotional-mind and physical-mind, and identify falsehoods masquerading as truth. Open the lotus in the heart and bring peace forward.

5. Seek a higher view—a life affirming view.
   Ask without hidden motive and be surrounded by your answer. Name the wrong understanding from a physical, emotional/somatic, mental, and spiritual standpoint, and by stepping back, affirm life-giving and health-enhancing options.

6. Set new intentions using intuition and vision.

Aim for the integral, intracognitive transcendence that, like a magnet-draws, heart-mind, inspiration, and intuitive vision.

7. Activate a healing response.

Focus consciousness, right attitude of mind, forgiveness, and faith; release all obstructions and name and reframe perceptions; and accompany them with supportive emotional responses and a renewed faith in Self and soul.

8. Build an integral healing plan within the context of your 'readiness' today.

Know your 'index of readiness', enlist the sacred patience that attracts the higher knowledge and repels ignorance, and nurture gratitude.

9. Establish checkpoints and choice-points.

Utilize witness consciousness combined with aspiration and a willingness to reject with heightened discernment; this will keep the checkpoints and choice-points in the foreground.

10. Affirm the repatterning processes that resolve your issue and related issues, and build faith in your soul-centered aspiration as you redesign your future.

Seek a soul-centered, happy, and peaceful heart; an awake and aware thought-mind that is engaged and vigilant; and an aligned higher emotional-vital. Allow your innate physical natural healing abilities to unfold.

15
Rebirth and Karma

The theory of rebirth is almost as ancient as thought itself and its origin is unknown. We may according to our prepossessions accept it as the fruit of ancient psychological experience always renewable and verifiable and therefore true or dismiss it as a philosophical dogma and ingenious speculation; but in either case the doctrine, even as it is in all appearance well-nigh as old as human thought itself, is likely to endure as long as human beings continue to think....Reincarnation is the popular term, but the idea in the word leans to the gross or external view of the fact and begs many questions. I prefer 'rebirth', for the Sanskrit term, punarjanma, 'again-birth' and commits us to nothing but the fundamental idea which is the essence and the life of the doctrine.
-Sri Aurobindo (Ghose, 1991, p.3).

Time and time again, Sri Aurobindo encourages us to pull free from the tamasic need to simplify, to make black and white, to decrease complexity, and to decree with simple statements—blinding ourselves to the vast and inspiring nature of this multidimensional existence. Wisdom, he reiterates, comes with the simultaneous development of heart and mind. Wisdom does not lie in narrowness, in a shallow grave of right and wrong—it lies in wideness and depth, guided by an awakened psychic being or soul awareness and by a heightened healthy egoic, or better, Beyond-ego awareness. In this chapter we share only a small part of the Integral yoga teachings on rebirth and karma as it informs this perspective on human becoming.

The soul, Sri Aurobindo says, determines the rebirth:

> The psychic being at the time of death chooses what
> it will work out in the next birth and determines the
> character and conditions of the new personality.
> Life is for the evolutionary growth by experience in
> this condition of the Ignorance till one is ready for
> the higher Light. (Ghose, 1999, p. 135)

He encourages us to view death as a process, one guided
by more than the shadow aspects of our fear or even the
terror that surrounds this time of bodily leaving. We have
a purpose here on earth that we may or may not fulfill, but
our time of leaving—our transition—comes with a renewed
sense of the role of the Eternal. In *Savitri*, he writes:

> Although Death walks beside us on Life's road,
> A dim bystander at the body's start
> And a last judgment on man's futile works,
> Other is the riddle of its ambiguous face;
> Death is a stair, a door, a stumbling stride
> The soul must take to cross from birth to birth,
> A grey defeat pregnant with victory,
> A whip to lash us toward our deathless state.
> The inconscient world is the spirit's self-made room,
> Eternal Night shadow of eternal Day.
> Night is not our beginning nor our end;
> She is the dark Mother in whose womb we have hid
> Safe from too swift a waking to world-pain.
> We came to her from a supernal Light,
> By Light we live and to the Light we go.
> (Ghose, 2005, Book X, canto 1, pp. 600-601).

Though mostly veiled from our daily existence, the soul is
in training, attempting to master the evolutionary process
on behalf of each individual, of humankind, and moreover,
of the Universal plan. He tells us that the old Vedantins
were not so enamored of the personality; they saw a
continuity of Self, a persistent immortal Self reflected in a
flowing river of change (Ghose, 1991). The causal, astral,
and subtle strings of Consciousness, Force, Energy, Light,

and Information are what connect to the central channel and the chakras, providing life- force and a soul wisdom to our heart-strings. The strings of Consciousness initiate the innermost being, then the inner being, and finally, our personality-based outer being however fractured, changing, or integrated it may be.

This incarnation, Sri Aurobindo shares, is to "find and fulfill consciously the universal being's hidden significance [that] is the task given to the human spirit" (Ghose, 1991, p. 44). In other words, each rebirth provides individuals with an opportunity to access soul and unfold spiritual purpose as a gift of grace to humankind and to all beings; ongoing transcendent Becoming is thus a cause and a purpose for rebirth. He continues: "We are a soul of the transcendent Spirit and Self unfolding itself in the cosmos" (p. 44). Each human has a higher role and a purpose; however, there is mystery connected with the riddle that holds the secret of the Way deep in the bosom of the Divine.

Part of the secret of rebirth can be described in the form of Karma. After much discernment and after studying many traditions of karma, Sri Aurobindo suggested a viewpoint that is interwoven into our perspective here. He elucidates four pillars of karma that present a theory about how Self and Nature interlink over time and space.In the first pillar of karma,

> there is an ordered Energy at work which assures its will by law and fixed relation and steady succession and links of ascertainable cause and effectuality. To be assured that there is an all-pervading mental law and all- pervading moral law...[therefore] what I sow in the proper soil, I shall assuredly reap...But there is a possibility that if this Energy is all, I may only be a creation of an imperative Force and all my acts and becomings a chain of determination over which I can have no real control of chance of mastery. (Ghose, 1991, p. 73).

This pillar offers a nice, tidy resolution, with everything attributable to predestination. Sri Aurobindo tells us that this outcome might satisfy our intellect "...but it would be disastrous to the greatness of my spirit. I would be a slave and puppet of Karma and could never dream of being a sovereign of myself and my existence" (p. 74).

Second, he outlines an idea that works with relations and creates relations: "...by will, the energy of the Idea in me develop[s] the form of what I am and arrive[s] at the harmony of some greater idea that is expressed in my present mould and balance. I can aspire to a nobler expansion" (Ghose, 1991, p. 74). However, this Idea cannot stand alone—it must be connected to something more certain and more in harmony with a universal order. This pillar begins the process of self-mastery.

For the third pillar, there is an admission

that I am a soul developing and persisting in the paths of the universal Energy and that in myself is the seed of all my creation. What I have become, I have made myself by the soul's past idea and action, its inner and outer karma; what I will to be, I can make myself by present and future idea and action. (Ghose, 1991, p. 74).

Here, we see the reference to involution and evolution taking effect.

The fourth pillar is even more liberating: "both the Idea and its Karma may have their origin in the free spirit and by arriving at myself by experience and self-finding I can exalt my state beyond all bondage of karma to spiritual freedom" (Ghose, 1991, p. 74).

This pillar of karma relies on the involutionary and evolutionary process—on the willingness of individuals to shake free of the hold of tamas and of the mechanical, easily wooed, and trance-like rote ways of being as well as of the blameful and outward projection of all shame, anger, guilt, or justifications for greed. This action includes releasing the neediness that can never be assuaged, the habits that become engrained before deeper reflection has given a true acceptance, the despair that sits at our doorstep when we firmly believe it ought not to given our abundance, and even the sadness and fear that creates deeper and deeper grooves of helplessness. There must be more—and in the most terrific and horrific of human conditions, some have found this 'more'.

We have seen that letting Nature have its way with the emotional-vital and the lower levels of mind does not serve the soul or the higher spiritual faculties. The old, habitual ways of the 'old me' can create a hell on earth— for many, if not a certain hell then an emptiness of the inner vessel. Material possessions and rajastic behavior or violation just cannot fill that emptiness for more than a moment. If rajastic behavior is determinedly pushed beyond reason, catching individuals in its net, the lower forces build and create greater havoc that takes the person back to black, back to the shadow, and back to the rule of the subconscient and unconscious forces: the war zone. Who is in charge then? Some thoughts on this question are included in the epilogue.

The raw materials for rebirth and karma combine our present personality and egoic characteristics; heredity from the physical, emotional-vital, mental, and spiritual perspectives; environmental forces; past lifetime lessons; learning; and the aim of the higher Self and spirit for this lifetime. Sri Aurobindo tells us that rebirth is the

> continuity of that self-effectuation in the individual, the persistence of the thread; Karma is the process, a force, a work of energy and consequence in the material world, an inner and outer will, an action and mental, moral, dynamic consequence in the soul evolution of which the material world is the constant scene. (Ghose, 1991, p. 100).

Karma is far more than a plus and minus system set in place irrevocably—it is complex and not easily understood even by the great masters. Karma is action, with a doer and a consequence: hence, the inner and outer being in their mighty collisions of dynamic movement are involved. There are consequences from all angles for each of the planes of being: physical, emotional-vital, and mental for ranges of ideation; and moral as well as spiritual. All consequences, no matter how small, have these angles. Moreover, underlying each activity is a will from Nature, a call from above and a still small voice perhaps from the soul. Furthermore, there are dimensions far beyond even the most erudite yogi's abilities to ascertain, interfacing and co-creating a process beyond our ken.

Our life is a field of action, and evolution is consciously (or not) the aim for us. We can engage in a process of self- finding and self-mastery by widening, deepening, and broadening our conscious awareness, and by awaking to a witness consciousness that realizes the creative gift and mystery that lie within the great Brahman or Universal transcendent. We can accept our part through the right use of aspiration, rejection, and surrender and through a wise tempering of the gunas.

Karma is an instrument of growth; when taken individually and globally, our lessons (part of the earth-school), our pains, and our sorrows ask something of humanity. A larger numinous plan is at work, and we—lifetime after lifetime—take our turn abiding within the Spirit's plan and the soul's agenda, with the freedom to awaken and more consciously own our actions and our contribution to humankind as well as to this beautiful planet that hosts us.

Sri Aurobindo assures us that there is no clear cut and simple formula for karma; there is choice and a many-sided oneness (Ghose, 1991). However, Professor Arabinda Basu offers a blunt and easier theme to start in a translation of the parable *Swapna* from its original Bengali. In it, Sri Aurobindo provides an explanation for the Law of Karma: "Not reward or punishment— but the creation of evil from evil, good from good. This is a natural law. Sin is evil, from that is suffering, virtue is good, from that comes happiness"

(Basu, 1995, p. 44). Taken literally, this statement provides a place to start, but not to close. As we have seen, this statement has multiple complexities and nuances when viewing the human being from an evolutionary framework.

We turn now to our final chapter: lighting the flame.

16
Human Becoming:
Lighting the Flame of Inquiry

Where do we go from here? Integral yoga asks us to raise the depth and breadth of our consciousness and to heighten our sensitivity—our awareness—and our ability to awaken. We are asked to bring down stillness and truth steeped in wisdom: to take the Path of Ascent, by widening and deepening our consciousness, and by bringing stillness and receptive silence. This, we are told, opens the doors to the Path of Descent, of receiving from higher mind or spiritual-mind wisdom and of enabling wisdom to well up from the soul-center within.

This book places the yogic science of Sri Aurobindo at our doorstep. Human becoming is something different for everyone, and Integral yoga as it is elucidated here provides an aim and guidelines for life change and soul growth. Sri Aurobindo and the Mother's quotes share their clear view, the research material with quotes from practitioners and clients alike presents a lived view from in-the-moment, Julia's story shares portions of one individual's awakening, and all are woven into a perspective that we hope takes the research and reflective practices further and provides an educational guideline for self-reflection.

Before any personal or lasting meaningful change, there must be aspiration—a flame of inquiry birthed within the individual. Crucially, as we have seen, for real change to occur there must be a willingness to make an effort, to aspire, and to support internal processes that (a) compassionately and actively repair fractured ego-states; (b) nurture lessons learned from the subpersonalities; (c) integrate the subpersonalities while guided gently by the deeper sacred heart and kindly by the thought-mind; (d) allow the higher-emotional-vital, higher mind, and spiritual mind to be inspired; and (e) seek the soul-openings that nurture the Beyond ego. This is no easy task. The Mother says; "The easy path generally leads nowhere" (Dalal, 2002, p. 78).

How do we attain personhood and a wise, healthy, strong, centralized, and discerning ego? How can we address our own demons and shadow-selves, our lower selves, our anger, despair, craving, and the multiple wants that are not true needs? How do we stand steadfast during moments or days of despair? How do we quietly (or not) and with integrity contribute to our community and our nation? How can we ensure that we have a nurturing impact on global humankind—an impact that respectfully sustains the Integral yoga mission of unity in diversity. Is this possible? Who answers? How many answers are there? How do we start to even find an answer? How do we know we have even started?

From Sri Aurobindo's yoga the need is clear to enlarge and raise the consciousness of being—to direct human becoming. There is no escape from waking existence, but there are infinite ways to be awake, from the most tranced mechanical, to the states that mark the highly sensitive leaders supporting human rights and global cooperation, to the quietly wise and courageous individuals of every nation.

How do we learn to hold hope for ourselves and others when we understand that evolution does not follow a straight path? It follows a spiralling path whereby one reaches a peak and then dips down to heal new aspects of the self that are now ready, and then as they are healed, the spiral climbs again but higher—the valley, no matter how deep, has to be traversed for the next height to appear. This process takes faith steeped in understanding. Nevertheless, without a healthy ego, it is formidable if not impossible to attain self-mastery of a process such as this. Centralizing the ego and keeping it healthy enough is paramount.

This chapter discusses Sri Aurobindo's four great instruments that can be used to sustain the practice of yoga: *shastra*, the knowledge of truths; *utsasha*, the force of personal effort; *guru*, the influence of the Inner Guide and perhaps an outer teacher to sustain the personalized effort; and *kala*, the instrumentality of Time (Ghose, 1996). These instruments have a two-fold agenda: they assist the conscious aspect of evolution, and while encouraging the development of thought-mind and the higher emotional-vital, they also nurture processes that go beyond ego and elevate to spiritual-mind and higher-mind processes, engendering a soul-centered depth.

Shastra is learning the truths, principles, powers, and processes governing the inner and outer activities that nurture access to the soul. In Integral yoga, the eternal Veda is within, centered in the innermost being of each individual as a bud—a lotus, folded up and closed in the innermost being. Human becoming is the unfolding of this bud set deep within the innermost being. The process is one of self-knowledge and an increasing awakening or unfolding of consciousness. The knowledge can come from the sacred texts that provide foundations; however, in many places Sri Aurobindo advocates going beyond the text. All shastra, he says, is developed from the past to help the future, but only as an aide and partial guide. Equally, much depends on personal effort and upon the power of the Inner Guide (Ghose, 1996).

The force of personal effort, utsasha is initially required to centralize the ego and bring forth a healthy, integrated personality capable of exceeding itself and opening naturally to the transcendent. Personal effort in the form of aspiration is required to turn the direction of the thought-mind upward and the higher emotional-vital inward. This tapasaya requires a power of the heart, a force of the will, and concentration of the mind combined with perseverance and determination, and interwoven with faith in this ancient experience outlined in the great spiritual traditions tapasya. Here, healthy ego is the instrument then learning a complex and intricate process of going Beyond ego. As we have seen, the effort is considerable— as are the rewards.

Guru refers to the influence of the Guide: As noted the supreme shastra is the eternal Veda, the secret wisdom in the heart of each person, so the supreme guru is the Inner Guide once the soul has been awakened (Ghose, 1996). The light of this knowledge brings a direct knowing of wisdom and intimations of the right path. The aim is to get beyond the ego, beyond one's own illusions, beyond all the material the outer being throws in the way, and beyond the social, environmental, and subtle astral impediments. The work is to contact one's highest Self, soul, or the highest Self in all. Sri Aurobindo assures us that even though the ego cannot understand and may revolt or lose confidence or courage, the Divine is not offended by our failures or weaknesses—the Divine holds great love and great patience. However, if we withdraw our consent, we lose the conscious awareness that gives us intimations of a greater assistance (Ghose, 1996, 2000c). It is we who get restless, who wish to be dazzled, who succumb to subtle trance states or glamor—this type of ignorance can turn to disaster: but once the aspiration returns, this ignorance can be turned again toward inner awakening, reaffirming a self-admitted willingness to step forth. The natural call to the soul brings a true meaning to life—and then the work, a responsible and self-aware tapasya, takes a new turn.

Lastly, Kala or Time as instrument removes the time-pressure from daily existence. This path, birth and death, and rebirth are intertwined in a sacred process (Sri Aurobindo, see Ghose, 1991). We can make time an enemy or a friend; we can resist it, or term it a medium or an instrument. To the ego, Time is a tyrant, and to the Divine an instrument. It is our choice— there is much freedom here and we can use the mind to make time a friend.

Each of these four instruments or aids in the yoga can be used as the outer-being consciousness becomes more and more integrated. In particular, the outer-being consciousness becomes more in touch with the inner-being ranges of subliminal influence, the social and environmental aspects of life, and most important, the innermost, soul-centered wisdom resting behind the veil.

With the understandings offered here and complemented by additional inward and outward seeking, a greater sense of self and soul can be established internally. As Sri Aurobindo assures us, Integral yoga uses all of who we are—all of what we have done, thought, dreamed, and fantasized (Ghose, 1996, 2000c). If we are willing and bring forth our aspiration, our willingness to reject the lower-self call and the emotional-vital wanderings and beliefs that take us off course, if we use aspiration in a patient, calm, and sattwic manner—then we can overcome, change, and find a process of sadhana and soul-centered living that fits our degree of readiness. Moreover, we can find joy in the journey because it is the journey of our life, our svabhava dharma, bringing our meaning and purpose forward and holding the light for ourselves, our family, our community, our nation, and global humankind. With grace, we can actively accept our part of the unity in diversity: to unfold consciousness, receive the light, energy, force, and information that is ours to claim and to share. This is the process of human becoming.

A sincere aspiration that is wide enough and deep enough to embody the highest Consciousness, Force, Energy, Light, and Information—this sources the mysterious and numinous aspects of human becoming. Moreover, and with this context in mind, Sri Aurobindo scholar and yogi Seidlitz (2008-2009) advocates:

> We must learn to always depend on the Divine, calling on its help and intervention. The knowledge and power of the Divine are omniscient and

omnipotent, and if we resolutely put ourselves in its hands, surrendering to its will and action, we can be sure of our successful navigation through all the trials and difficulties of the Yoga, to the supreme deliverance and transformation (p. 19).

We part with these words from Sri Aurobindo (Ghose, 2005, p. 476):

> "Remember why you cam'st:
> Find out thy soul, recover thy hid self..."

It is summer as I write the final chapters of this text (2011). News of riots in London, England hit the press as does that of ongoing repression in several Middle Eastern countries, of famine in Somalia, and of the dept crisis in Europe and the United States. Even the city we live in had its own riots in the Spring of this year following the hockey playoffs, with millions of dollars of damage in the city core. (Interestingly, 47 of the 1,115 people the police sought turned themselves in—even they did not want to become like the plunderers they had joined for a few thoughtless moments). Radiation from the Japanese Fukiyama plant destroyed after the earthquake and tsunami continues to pour radiation into the air, earth, and ocean, and we hear very differing accounts of how much radiation. Recently, a whole police force resigned in a Mexican border town.

This list, I realize, hardly touches other news of equal intensity. Is there a continent or country untouched by aspects of trouble?

Conversely, is there a country whose leaders are responsibly managing its affairs with integrity, taking their sacred stewardship of the land and people, and their global responsibilities in stride in ways that sustain support of the thinking and clear-minded citizenry?

I wondered: What if I applied the notion of war zone consciousness as it was initiated in my earlier research, developed in this text, and further refined as I contemplated the impact of this rendition of Integral yoga's map of consciousness.

A definition for our purposes:

War Zone consciousness *is the battle that takes place when rational and even wisdom-based supra-rational consciousness, inner awareness, and considered common sense battle with powerful emotional-vital forces such as rage, anger, despair, greed, vanity, graspings for power, and a myriad of illusory shallow, shadow, and narrow belief sets leading to raging, out-of-control, emotionally driven behaviors. Malevolently, these very heightened and intensified negative emotions attract forces from the subtle and astral worlds. Far more destructive and often brilliant and cunning or depraved and cunning, these forces start to intervene in human consciousness. Individuals are soon overtaken, becoming instruments of an ugliness beyond comprehension. In these instances the still-small voice-of-the-soul is left far behind, shrouded and shrivelled. Common sense is hijacked. The inner and higher knowing of those involved, while awake at differing levels of their being, is nonetheless appalled.*

Intimidation (whether subtle or not) and a sense of helplessness, often engendered by individuals and groups with political, media, and corporate agendas, can both ignite the path of destruction—for the individual as well as the city or state. Moreover, the exact people who lead and influence the politics, media mandates, and corporate lobbying are no different; they too can be driven instruments of powers they admit based on their own weaknesses. However, having accepted leadership positions, they are more culpable because they are more aware (or perhaps callously, uncaringly, unaware) of their driven agendas and more expansively manipulative in how they use their power.

Senior fellow of The National Institute and award-winning journalist Chris Hedges (2009) writes:

Our nation has been hijacked by oligarchs, corporations, and a narrow, selfish, political, and economic elite, a small privileged group that governs, and often steals, on behalf of moneyed interests. This elite, in the name of patriotism and democracy, in the name of all the values that were once part of the American [USA] system and defined the Protestant work ethic, has systematically destroyed our manufacturing sector, looted our treasury, corrupted our democracy, and trashed our financial system. During this plundering we remain passive, mesmerized by the enticing shadows on the wall, assured our ticket to success, prosperity and happiness were waiting around the corner. The government, stripped of any real sovereignty, provides little more than technical expertise for elites and corporations that lack moral restraints and a concept of the common good (p. 142- 143).

Is this only true of the United States? I suspect from what I read that Hedges speaks of a global mindset, and hence a fearsome global state of affairs. With an Integral yogic perspective as this text discusses: Who is in charge—really? Once individuals become corrupt and the corruption becomes endemic, as the ancients have tried to tell us for centuries, there are unseen forces that live on the food of destruction— they seek fuel, and as hungry ghosts they are never full. Their promise is to ultimately destroy those who succumb—the citizenry—as well as those they rule and play with as their puppets. Indeed, powerful, well educated rulers of our land are equally susceptible because power, money, and even sex hold keys that call in enticements.

Unless individuals are principled and strong in character, have a healthy ego, and are capable of accessing the wisdom of the sacred heart, they can most easily sell their soul to the lower forces. How many leaders do we have, in any capacity, who care enough to see the bigger picture or who consciously agree to walk wisely and courageously with integrity? Who supports them?

Leading historian Tony Judt (2010), reflects:

> Something is profoundly wrong with the way we live today. For thirty years we have made a virtue out of the pursuit of material self-interest: indeed, this very pursuit now constitutes whatever remains of our sense of collective purpose. We know what things cost but have no idea what they are worth. We no longer ask of a judicial ruling or a legislative act; is it good? Is it fair? Is it just? Is it right? Will it bring about a better society or a better world? Those used to be the political questions, even if they invited no easy answers. We must learn once again to pose them (p. 1-2).

The young people want to ask exactly these questions. However, after teaching in academic programs for years, Judt notes:

> Indeed the rising generation is acutely worried about the world it is to inherit. But accompanying these fears there is a general sentiment of frustration: 'we' know something is wrong and there are many things we don't like. But what can we believe in? What should we do? (pp. 3-4).

It will take more than a sound, rational mind to turn this ship of materialism, consumerism, and dept toward a new goal— yet it can be done. Historically, it is has been done. Someone somewhere has to stop promising the false 'magic bullet' to right the economic, corporate, and political wrongs, and stop capitulating to those who lobby for the political wrongs. Someone has to declare that it is wrong to pander to the stock market and increasingly criminalize dissent that comes from sensible, kind, and thoughtful thinking citizens; indeed, denying them and promoting state-encouraged selfishness is wrong. Someone has to call the governments on their false expenses, false monetary policies, premeditated false use of language tactics, false adjustments now called 'hedonistic adjustments' of

statistics (e.g., the inflation index), management of our
monies for the betterment of the banks, management of
our health for the betterment of the pharmaceutical and
high tech companies, and more.

Someone somewhere has to convince the public
who are now becoming walking drug prescriptions. What
is concerning, certainly in the West, is that more adults
and children are turning to psychotropic medications,
and youth to illegal drugs. But drugging stress and anxiety
away is not the solution; a dazed, sedated, numbed half-
mind and half-body eventually racked by side-effects is
not the answer. A wide awake, calm, and thinking citizenry
is needed now more than ever—as this text attests, and
Hedges (2009), Judt (2010), and many other brave authors
and journalists from many countries succinctly report.

Only with a calm, clear mind and a hope for humanity
can individuals identify the intentionally inflammatory
political rhetoric used by politicians and the media who
support them; only then can individuals notice how
language is abused. Double- speak crassly abounds and is
well used by politicians, the military, and in advertising; all
aim at triggering (subtly or not) the lower-emotional-vital
fear, greed, or dissatisfaction in the use of words or tone.
Individuals are encouraged to believe one thing and subtly
(or not) convinced to refuse to entertain another view.

Certainly this is not the time to be coerced into
believing that the state, the banks, or the increasingly giant
and mega- budget corporations hold the secret to success
or can withstand even a modicum of serious scrutiny. Only
those citizens who are wide awake and capable of thinking
for themselves will recognize when these very entities in
their broadcasts, publications, or advertising are pandering
to emotional-vital lower aspects. Media may feed them the
hate or fear that maybe a small part of them does crave—
or, on the other hand, may oh- so-gently dish out soma,
an illusory and nice-sounding cocktail of trance-inducing
comfort.

Only awake and aware individuals will recognize when they have been caught in tribal warfare, one group against another group, and both groups have now become small minded, angry, and greedy. And for what? The good of society as a whole? Surely most thinking people have a sense of what basically can work for their home, their country, and the globe. Why not have dialogue—a dialogue steeped in stewardship, vision, and sound business practices, with well orchestrated morally and ethically sound leadership. This type of dialogue taps into the heritage of human wisdom and human hope, reaches far beyond to the deepest heart-knowing, and activates the supra-rational mind where creative ideas and ideals reside.

Sri Aurobindo speaks of a vision of the future:

> The coming of a spiritual age must be preceded by the appearance of an increasing number of individuals who are no longer satisfied with the normal intellectual, vital and physical existence of man, but perceive that a greater evolution is the real goal of humanity and attempt to effect it in themselves, to lead others to it and to make it the recognized goal of the race. In proportion as they succeed and to the degree to which they carry this evolution, yet the unrealised potentiality which they represent will become an actual possibility of the future. (Ghose, 1997, p. 263)

Individuals can join together in small groups and take ownership of societal issues and themes. They can present wise counsel and contribute to the political agenda on many fronts. For example, they can inform healthcare professionals that pathologizing is not to be used for the whole population, carte blanche manipulated as a decree—instead, pathology identified accurately and treated well is only for those with genuine disorders identified by proven scientific testing results. Good science is not pathologizing our mental health creating ever larger *Diagnostic and*

Statistical Manuals of Mental Disorders, and certainly can only serve the billion-dollar prescription industry. Lifestyle changes, concrete wellness strategies, and a health-engendering society with consumer activism offer a far more proactive answer.

Known as a radical historian, the late Howard Zinn (2009) cautions against the despair that can come from noting endless cycles of deception, endless cycles of retaliation, escalating endless cycles of terrorism (subtle and overt), and the fall-out of moral nakedness. In his writings he assures us (as does Sri Aurobindo, see Ghose, 2000c) that truth comes out—its power is greater than lies and deception. He advocates that individuals join heart and mind, refuse stupidity, raise hard questions, and take action: Do something to create a better world.

Taking action can include asking wellness-based healthcare professionals and educators to ply us all at the earliest ages and on into adulthood with lifestyle and sophisticated consciousness-based wellness tools for success. Such tools can address our overall wellbeing: the physical, emotional/somatic, mental, and spiritual as well as the social and environmental nature of human existence, and at levels that leave much room for creativity, multicultural nuances, and personal choice. Let us look at this planet and find a job-for-all, including volunteering; let us find hope-for-all; and let us seek the deeply meaningful purpose that lies hidden behind human existence and behind the creation of this beautiful planet.

Sri Aurobindo reminds us that "unity is as strong a principle of which division is only a subordinate term, and to the principle of unity every divided form must therefore subordinate itself" (Ghose, 1990, p. 215). This is a dynamic unity in diversity—a valuing of freedom governed by an overarching complex view of the planet as a whole, with each person uniquely contributing and each being as wise as possible in the moment. In this unity, each person can hold those who are graced with leadership in the countries that consciously and sincerely participate to a higher, truer, courageous, insightful, wisely principled, and compassionate co-creative stewardship of humankind and the planet as a whole.

May it be so.

REFERENCE SELECTION

Alfassa, M. (The Mother). (1998). *Health and healing in yoga* Pondicherry, India: Sri Aurobindo Ashram Trust.

Alfassa, M. (The Mother). (2003). *Words of long ago.* Pondicherry, India: Sri Aurobindo Ashram Trust.

Alfassa, M. (The Mother). (2005). *Prayers and meditations* Pondicherry, India: Sri Aurobindo Ashram Trust.

Bakshi, G.D. (1999). *Kundalini.* Varanasi, India: Pilgrims Publishing

Basu, A. (1995). *Questions and answers.* Gavasena, Pondicherry, India: Sri Aurobindo Ashram.

Basu, A. (2011). *Unpublished transcript.* March, 2011.

Dalal, A. S. (2000). *Growing within.* Pondicherry, India: Sri Aurobindo Ashram Trust.

Dalal, A. S. (2001). *A greater psychology.* New York, NY: Tarcher/Putman.

Dalal, A. S. (2002). *Emergence of the psychic.* Pondicherry: Sri Aurobindo Ashram.

Dalal, A. S. (2007a). *Chakras, yoga-shakti and kundalini: Dynamics of spirit.* In Sri Aurobindo and the future of psychology (pp. 346-353). Pondicherry, India: Sri Aurobindo International Centre for Education.

Dalal, A. S. (2007b). *Our many selves. In Sri Aurobindo and the future of psychology* (pp. 198-213). Pondicherry, India: Sri Aurobindo International Centre for Education.

Dalal, A. S. (2007c). *Sri Aurobindo and the future psychology.* Pondicherry, India: Sri Aurobindo International Centre of Education.

Dispenza, J. (2007). *Evolve your brain.* Deerfield Beach, FL: Health Communications.

Doige, N. (2007). *The brain the changes itself.* London, England: Penguin Books.

Enginger, B. (Satprem). (1992). T*he mind of the cells.* Mount Vernon, WA: Institute for Evolutionary Research.

Ghose, A. (Sri Aurobindo). (1991). *Rebirth and karma.* Wilmot, WI: Lotus Light.

Ghose, A. (Sri Aurobindo). (1995). *Letters on yoga (Vol. 2).* Pondicherry, India: Sri Aurobindo Ashram.

Ghose, A. (Sri Aurobindo). (1996). *Synthesis of yoga.* Twin Lakes, WI: Lotus Light.

Ghose, A. (Sri Aurobindo). (1997). *The Human Cycle.* Pondicherry: Sri Aurobindo Ashram.

Ghose, A. (Sri Aurobindo). (1999). *The psychic being.* Pondicherry: Sri Aurobindo Ashram.

Ghose, A. (Sri Aurobindo). (2000a). *Letters on yoga (Vol. 1).*Pondicherry, India: Sri Aurobindo Ashram.

Ghose, A. (Sri Aurobindo). (2000b). *Letters on yoga (Vol. 3).* Pondicherry, India: Sri Aurobindo Ashram.

Ghose, A. (Sri Aurobindo). (2000c). *The life divine.* Twin Lakes, WI: Lotus Press.

Ghose, A. (Sri Aurobindo). (2004). Record of yoga (Vol. 1). Pondicherry, India: Sri Aurobindo Ashram.

Ghose, A. (Sri Aurobindo). (2005). *Savitri.* Pondicherry, India: Sri Aurobindo Ashram.

Ghose, A., & Alfassa, M. (Sri Aurobindo & the Mother). (2006). *Integral healing*. Pondicherry, India: Sri Aurobindo Ashram.

Ghose, A., & Alfassa, M. (Sri Aurobindo & the Mother). (1998). *A practical guide to Integral yoga*. Pondicherry, India: Sri Aurobindo Ashram.

Hedges, C. (2009). *Empire of illusion*. Toronto, Ontario, Canada: Alfred A. Knopf.

Johari, H. (2000). *Chakras: Energy centres of transformation*. Rochester, VT: Destiny Books.

Judt, T. (2010). *Ill fares the land*. London, England: Penguin Books.

Lamb, R. (2010). *Healing as yoga sadhana*. Ann Arbor, MI: Proquest (ublication no. AAT. 3405497.

Lipton, B., & Bhaerman, S. (2009). *Spontaneous evolution*. New York, NY: Hay House.

Miovic, M. (2007). *Sri Aurobindo and transpersonal psychology.* In A. S. Dalal (Ed)., *Sri Aurobindo and the future of psychology* (pp.11-49). Pondicherry, India: Sri Aurobindo Centre for Education.

Mother, the—see Alfassa.

Pandit, M. (1983). *Basis of sadhana*. Pondicherry, India: Dipiti. Pandit, M. P. (1992). Heart of sadhana. Pondicherry, India: Dipti.

Pandit, M. (1994). *The yoga of transformation*. Pondicherry, India: Dipti, Sri Aurobindo Ashram.

Pandit, M. (1999). *Yoga for the modern man*. Pondicherry, India: Sri Aurobindo Ashram.

Reddy, A. (2007). *Deliberations on the life divine.* Pondicherry,India: Sri Aurobindo Centre for Advanced Research.

Satprem—see Enginger.

Seidlitz, L. (2008/2009). *Practices in Integral Yoga.* Collaboration, 33(3), 11-19.

Sri Aurobindo—see Ghose.

Sri Aurobindo Ashram. (2004). *Integral healing.* Pondicherry, India: Sri Aurobindo Ashram Press.

Sri Aurobindo Ashram. (2006). *Towards perfect health.* Pondicherry, India: Sri Aurobindo Ashram Press.

Vannuci, M. (2005). *Integral yoga and psychoanalysis.* Genoa, Italy: Giotto.

Vrinte, J. (2002). *The perennial quest for psychology with a soul.* Delhi, India: Motilal Banarshidass.

White, J. (1990). *Kundalini evolution and enlightenment.* St. Paul, MN: Paragon House.

Woodroffe, J. (2006). Sakti and sakta. Madras, India: Ganesh & Co.

Zinn, H. (2009). *The Zinn reader.* New York, NY: Seven Stories Press.

Courses and Workshops

Dr. Lamb teaches courses based on this book as part of a college-based complementary health care certificate program, as well as courses open to the public. Participants have commented as follows:

• This course has inspired me to read more of Sri Aurobindo's teachings.
• Ruth does an amazing job of holding space and is very accessible/knowledgeable.
• Ruth is a knowledgeable teacher, her love of integral healing is obvious.
• Loved it, absolutely amazing...in awe of this course material.
• Excellent practices and information to enhance myself and so I can better assist others in their healing.
• This evolving program enhances my life journey; the deep inner connections are transformative.
• Thank you for having these fascinating and growth invoking courses.
• Exceptional integration of experiential components and cognitive theory.
• A unique pioneering transformational education experience.
• Very beautiful class on self-mastery.
• Extremely beneficial for self-awareness and great tools to use in professional practice.
• Beautiful facilitation, kind, gentle yet deeply intellectual.
• Exceptionally well prepared, condensed, and presented with appropriate experiential components.
• Exceptional program, provocative and powerful.
• Profound teachings; wonderful learning; personally life changing.
• I loved this course, it was great for understanding how and why people behave the way they do; I can now assist my clients in new ways.

About the Author

R.M. Lamb, Ph.D. works nationally and internationally with individuals, groups, and corporations interested in integral consciousness-based health promotion and self-empowerment approaches to well-being.

Following years of clinical practice, educational programming including curriculum design and teaching, and research, plus the study of complementary and alternative medicine, Dr. Lamb is contributing to the creation of a new paradigm of health care, a new paradigm of being-in-the-world, as she incorporates alongside ancient wisdom teachings.

For more information, please refer to the website:
www.cittamfutures.com

CPSIA information can be obtained at www.ICGtesting.com
Printed in the USA
LVOW04s2100110215

426641LV00028B/1369/P